Dedicated to those who lost their lives from breast cancer.

Acknowledgements

I would like to convey my personal thanks to all the sources from which I have gathered information. It is not possible to acknowledge individually – as there were too many sources. I am particularly grateful for the permission to reproduce the photographs from —

AstraZeneca UK Limited — For cover page.

Novartis Pharmaceuticals UK Ltd — For breast self-examination.

Ms. Sally Inch — Breast-feeding Adviser and Baby Friendly Co-ordinator — Oxford Branch of the Royal College of Midwives — for Lactational Mastitis and Breast-feeding posters.

Elsevier Science — Hand Book of Diseases of the Breast by Michael Dixon and Richard Sainsbury, First Edition - 1993, Page no. - 3,5,6,7,11,12, 56 & 86 (colour section).

British Medical Journal — Breast Reconstruction after Surgery — by J.D. Watson, J.R.C. Sainsbury, J.M. Dixon. BMJ - volume - 310 - issue no. 14th Jannuary 1995, Page no. - 118, 119 & 120.

A Manual of Clinical Surgery—by Dr. Somen Das. Fifth Edition, Fig. 30.4, 30.5 and 363.
(Clinical Method in Surgery—Old Book)

I am grateful to Dr. R. L. CHAWLA and Miss. S. MANDAL for their support, encouragement and sound criticism and Mr. N. BARBER for the preparation of the photographs.

I would also like to extend my thanks to Mr. Arun Bhattarcharjee and the staff of Swapna Printing for their hard work and helpful advice on planning and printing work. The list of thanks will not be complete without mentioning the name of Mr. S. N. Basu for his contribution in the whole operational process of this publication and Media Centre for distribution.

Dr. A. K. MANDAL.
Kolkata, December, 2002.

BREAST CARE
AWARENESS

By

Dr. A. K. MANDAL.

M.B.B.S.(CAL.), M.R.C.O.G.(LOND.).
Retired General Medical Practitioner.
AND
Ex. Clinical Assistant in the Department of Obstetrics
Mayday University Hospital, England.

Published by **Dr. A. K. MANDAL**
in KOLKATA - INDIA, December, 2002

Distributed by :

MEDIA CENTRE
261, A.P.C. Road, Kolkata - 700 006
Tel. : 2351-5515, Fax : 2225-5358

Contact :

E-mail : hapipaul@rediffmail.com **(For India)**

E-mail : amandal@gipsylon.freeserve.co.uk **(For Overseas)**

Printed at
Swapna Printing Works (P) Ltd.
Kolkata, India.

n – Year 200_

Cop. 02   A. K. MANDAL

Preface

This informative and comprehensive book aimed at readers of all ages and backgrounds, but in particular is targeted towards women in the reproductive and menopausal groups. Throughout the book an emphasis has been laid on the learning process. The aim to identify any problems sooner rather than later, and to take appropriate precautions to enjoy healthy and happy living. In the book certain repetitions was considered to be of sufficient importance to merit restatement in more than one occasion.

Dr. A. K. MANDAL
December, 2002

C O N T E N T S

CHAPTER 1

Breast Introduction

In every corner of the globe history shows that woman has a passion to love their own body because of the exciting changes, such as, physical, sexual, and emotional, which take place at different stages in their lives. These exciting changes not only alter their self-image but also make them more adventurous to learn and explore their own body. Among these changes, the development of the breast is the earliest and most rewarding and sensational one. The woman is always conscious about their figure, especially the breasts, because it identifies the female role. Hence the woman always admires her body in front of a mirror, whether dressed or undressed, relaxes and enjoys her body in a warm bath, and experiences pleasure and lively with others, especially with opposite sex.

At puberty, with the surge of sexual hormones, mainly oestrogen and progesterone, the development of the breast and the onset of menstrual period begins. The breast starts to develop step by step during this period and reaches its full glory during the pregnancy. It is very difficult to describe what constitutes normal size and shape of a breast. The normality depends on a variety of personal, racial, cultural and individual factors. The various shapes, such as, pear-shaped, conical, discoid, and hemispherical may have a genetic influence. In some parts of the world, a large breast represents signs of fertility, for example — Arabian and African countries, whereas in other parts small breasts are preferable especially to models and athletes — in Western countries. Drooping of the breasts may occur at any stage of a woman's life either due to a very large size and heaviness, or lack of fatty tissue and poor condition of the chest muscles (pectoralis major muscle). An unusual distorted shape due to strong binding or stretching may also have some cultural influence. Breasts normally, tend to become flaccid after a pregnancy and with age involutes unless replaced by fat. Biologically, it is the organ of milk secretion and designed for feeding infants.

The symmetrical size, shape, position and appearance of the breasts not only enhance a woman's own identity but also boost her morale. Thus a human breast can be described as a paired, fleshy, with doughy consistency and almost equal in size overlying on the fascia of the pectoralis major muscle on either side of the anterior chest wall.

CHAPTER 2

Breast Anatomy

The human breast is a cutaneous structure. The female breast is situated in the upper-anterior aspect of the chest wall, on either side, extending from the second to the sixth or seventh ribs and between the parasternal and pectoralis major muscles. Sometimes it may extend beyond the lateral border of the pectoralis major muscle towards the axilla as an axillary tail. The axillary tail is palpable in normal cases and more easily before a menstrual period and during lactation. A well-developed axillary tail sometimes causes confusion of a palpable lump or as an enlarged lymph node. Thus, it has a surgical importance.

The nipple is a conical protuberance in each breast, contains erectile tissue and is surrounded by a pigmented area called the areola. It is covered by thick and corrugated skin. At the apex lactiferous ducts open and in a naked eye it is very difficult to see these orifices because of these folds.

In a nulliparous woman, the nipple and areola are pink, especially in blondes whereas in a multiparous as well as in a brunette woman they are dark brown due to deposit of melanin pigment. The nipple contains both longitudinal and circular muscle fibres and supported by arteriovenous anastomosis. Thus, being an erectile structure, it points forwards and outwards, especially in response to stimulation.

The skin of the breast contains hair follicles, sebaceous glands and sweat glands. There are no hair follicles in the areola but near the periphery it contains morgagnis tubercles. The sebaceous glands underneath the areola called montgomerys glands, enlarge during pregnancy and lubricate the nipple during lactation and open its duct on the surface of montgomerys tubercle.

In a fully developed breast, there are 15 to 20 lobes separated from one another by interlobular septa converging at the nipple. Each lobe is irregularly lobulated and has its own main duct, which opens, on the nipple. These ducts branch out in to terminal tubules, which end in alveoli. The alveoli are surrounded by myoepithelial contractile network, which also covers the ducts. Immediately before opening on the nipple each duct had a little reservoir for milk, called terminal ampulla preceded by a larger lactiferous sinus. These sinuses lie immediately beneath the areola.

The breasts are richly supplied with several blood vessels such as, internal mammary artery and lateral thoracic artery and acromiothoracic artery as well as lymph capillaries. As in other parts of the body, the lymph capillaries are connected with the lymph capillaries of the neighbouring structures of the opposite side and of the abdominal wall and thus play an important role in the spread of malignant disease.

Developmental abnormality of the breast can be seen from time to time, though less than five percent of the population, as a supernumerary or accessory nipple or as a supernumerary or accessory breast.

The accessory nipples are commonly noticed just below the normal breast along the milk line, whereas the accessory breast tissue are seen at the lower part of the axilla. Normally, they do not require any treatment unless they are causing psychological upset or unsightly.

Occasionally, absence of one breast can also be seen but it is often in associated with defect in the pectoralis muscle.

Asymmetry of the breast is norm rather than exception—the left breast is usually slightly larger than the right breast. The main reasons for asymmetry of the breast are due to the development of any tumour, injury or following a treatment of surgery or radiotherapy.

Breast asymmetry can be corrected either by augmentation or by reduction or by lifting the larger breast or by a combination of the procedures accordingly.

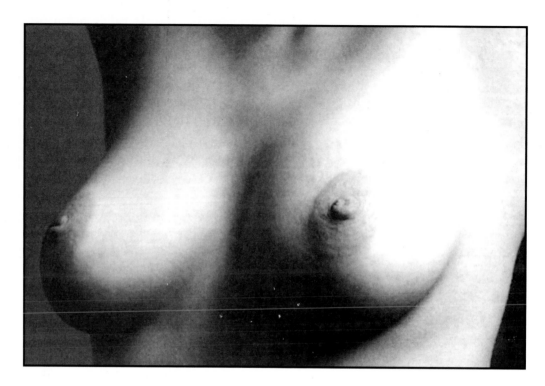

Adult breast

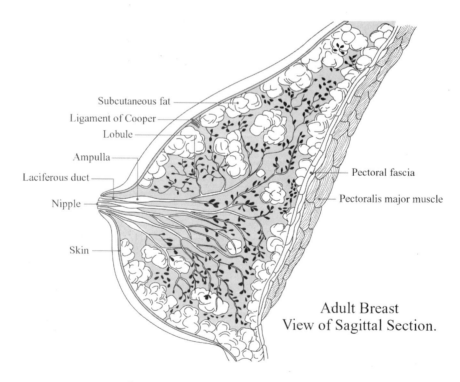

Subcutaneous fat
Ligament of Cooper
Lobule
Ampulla
Laciferous duct
Nipple
Skin

Pectoral fascia
Pectoralis major muscle

Adult Breast
View of Sagittal Section.

Showing duct & lobulo-alveolar system.

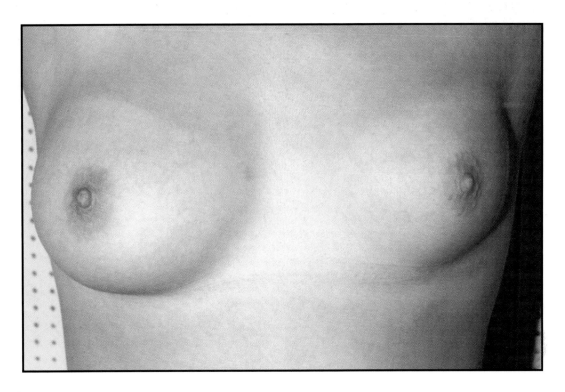

Inequality of the breast

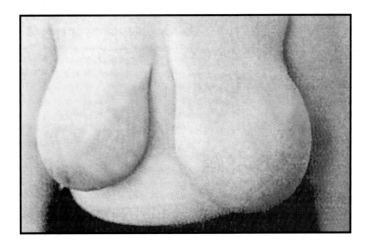

Large breasts

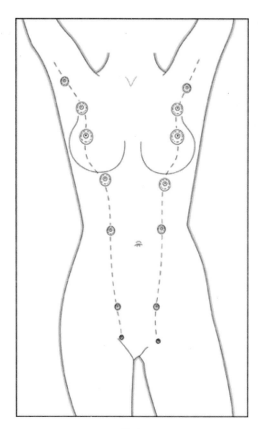

Milk line

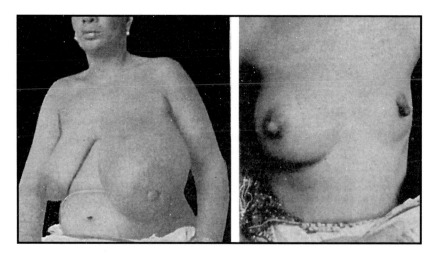

Hypertrophy and atrophy of the left breasts

(Permission given to reproduce this photograph - by Dr. S. Das)

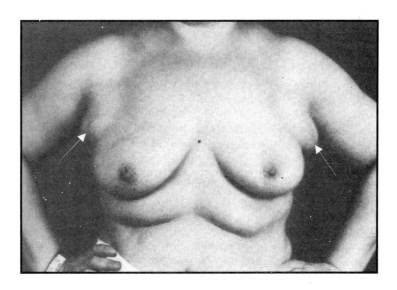

Patient with bilateral axillary accessory breasts

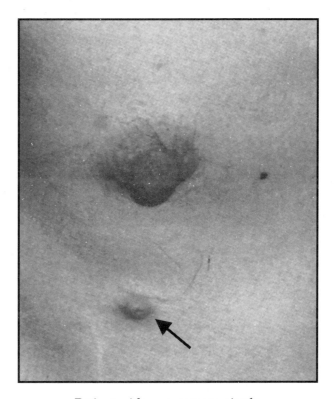

Patient with an accessory nipple.

CHAPTER 3

Breast Physiological Changes

At birth, the breast consists of a flattened nipple, a rudimentary duct system, myoepithelial cells, connective tissue epithelium and little glandular tissue. The nipple and areola are pigmented. The branch likes' duct system from each segment converges to form a single duct, which opens on the nipple. In a new- born infant a small nodule can be felt below both nipples and a milk secretion called colostrum milk (witches' milk) may be expressed from the nipples from the fourth to seventh postpartum day. The secretion may last for three to four weeks and is due to stimulation of placental hormones. At this stage, any increase in breast size is mainly due to increase in fat and connective tissue. Normally, after the first neonatal month the breast tissues regress and disappear after six months.

As puberty approaches, with the surge of sex hormones, mainly oestrogen and progesterone, the female breasts gradually enlarge and acquire a feminine contour due to nipple prominence and deposition of fat. With the onset of menstruation and successive menstrual cycles, the ovarian oestrogen alone stimulates the growth and development of the duct system and lobular proliferation during each follicular and luteal phase of the menstrual cycle. Each menstrual cycle has a two part, the first part is called a proliferative or oestrogenic phase, while the second part is called the secretory phase with evidence of progesterone activity mainly in the glands.

During the pregnancy, the breast undergoes further maturation in preparation for lactation. The progesterone secreted by the ovary and placenta together with oestrogen causes considerable proliferation of the duct system and brings the alveoli to complete development. During the early part of pregnancy, there are fullness and tenderness in the breast, the nipple increases in size and becomes more sensitive and erectile and glands of montgomery become more prominent. The pigments are deposited around the areola (called a primary areola) and a few drops of clear fluid, called colostrum, may be squeezed out. Further growth of the mammary gland and proliferation of the lobulo-alveolar system occurs throughout the pregnancy and is mainly due to increased blood supply. In the last trimester, colostrum can be expressed from the breast but the lactation remains dormant.

During the puerperium, after the expulsion of the placenta, the pituitary secretion (prolactin) emerges and is influenced by the level of oestrogen whether it is low, high or balanced. Only a balanced oestrogen level stimulates an anterior pituitary gland to secrete prolactin, which is mainly responsible for milk secretion. The other hormones, corticosteroids and thyriod, play an important supportive role in breast development and lactation. Prolactin stimulates lactogenesis in the alveolar system, whereas oxytocin (also a pituitary hormone) initiates contraction of the myoepithelial cells. During the first 24 to 48 hours after the delivery, breast secretion called the colostrum is secreted followed by proper milk secretion. The colostrum is a yellowish fluid, containing fat globule, the colostrum corpuscles, and has a mineral, low sugar and moderate protein content. It is important to the infant because of high content of an antibody and lymphocytes and thus helps to protect against an un-sterile environment. Towards the end of the first week after birth, a considerable change in volume and character of the milk takes place. An adequate production of milk and maintenance of lactation depends on various factors, such as,

- well-developed lobulo-alveolar system with abundance of secretory tissue,
- the right number of hormones in right proportion,
- frequency and intensity of nipple stimulation by the suckling behaviour of the infant,
- the development and maintenance of neuroendocrine feed back mechanism and
- complete emptying of the alveoli and the duct.

Failure of any of these factors, either congenital or acquired, may be the basis of lactation failure. At the menopause, the breasts involute, the alveolus shrinks, the gland atrophies and hence the breasts loose their shape.

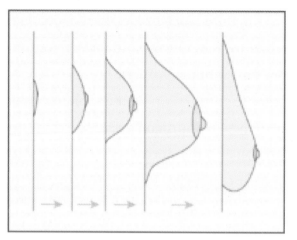

New born   Puberty   Adult   Menopause

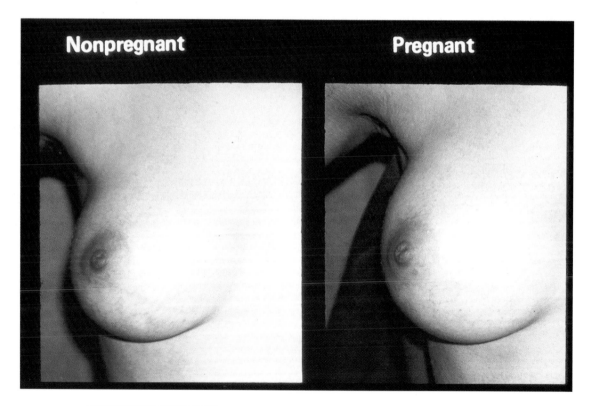

Nonpregnant   Pregnant

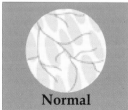

Normal

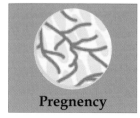

Pregnency

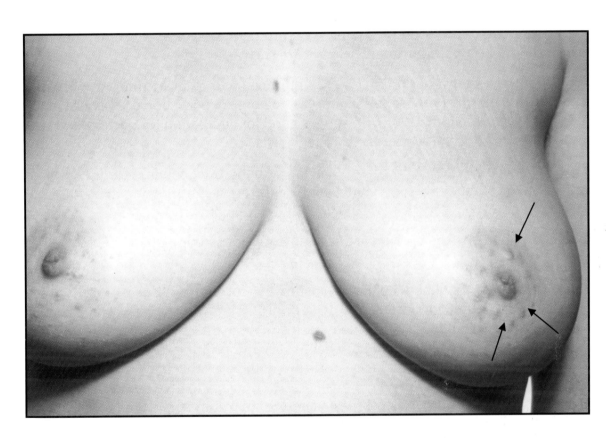

Prominent Montgomery's glands & cyst.

CHAPTER 4

Breast Care

Most of today's women are more body conscious than ever before. Women want to keep their whole body in shape by keeping a keen eye on their diet and exercise. Any forms of wrinkles and creases anywhere in the body, especially in the face and hands always take the priority on the list but the bust area is often unintentionally neglected. Like other areas of the body, a routine care of the breast is not only vital to physical and emotional well-being but also enhances the personal image, self-confidence and preserves their youthfulness in years to come. Regular breast maintenance should be a part of routine beauty care such as—

- regular exercises for a period of 15 to 20 minutes, two to three times a week as of brisk walking and specific exercise (for examples - elbow squeeze, box press, body bar lift, and moderately lightweight lifts). Swimming is good for circulation for pectoralis and shoulder muscles to improve the appearance of the breasts,

- a well-balanced diet consisting of protein, fat, carbohydrate, vitamins, minerals, fresh fruits and vegetables, etc. to avoid rapid weight gain or weight loss by controlling body fat collection,

- maintain a good posture to avoid artificial posture, as in stooping posture, to cover-up large breasts,

- regular check-up of vital statistics to ensure the correct size bra is worn with the best possible support and comfort. A poorly supporting bra can trigger various problems like itching from the bra hooks, and a smelly rash and often infection caused by sweating due to sagging breasts. Good all-round support is very important especially when exercising as well as breast-feeding. Now a day a sports bra with insertable pads that slip into the inside pocket of the bra top is available to push the bra upward to give a fuller effect. Similarly a maternity bra, especially when breast- feeding, plays an important role to support the breasts and thus avoid infection. The bra straps should be comfortable and adjustable and should be thick and wide enough to support the weight of the breasts,

- a regular examination (explained in self-breast examination chapter—5) of the breasts once in every month soon after the menstrual period while having either a bath or shower with warm soapy water or while laying flat in bed and

skin cares treatment, either by gel or ordinary body lotion or tonic or by simple face cream to moisturise in the breast area. If this area is exposed to ultraviolet rays especially during holidays, it undermines the collagen and elastin, and should be protected with a high factor sun cream.

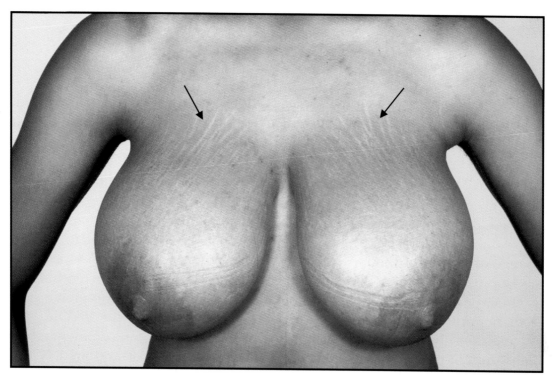

Hypertrophied (Pendulous) breasts — Note stretch marks

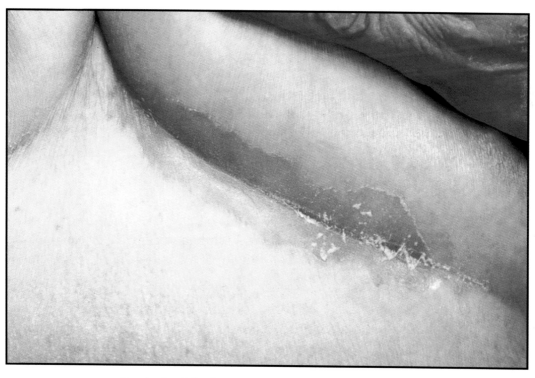

Psoriasis of the breast (under neath the large breast)

CHAPTER 5

Breast Self-examination

The aim of the self-examination of the breast is to enable a woman to detect and to notify any early changes in the breast to health professionals so that any disastrous effect can be minimised or corrected sooner rather than later. Age, desire to learn, social and educational background and even more important is the educational process itself, are the most important factors in the success of self-examination of the breasts. Despite recommendation of self-examination women were slow to complete the checks. Now, it is emerging that more and more women of different ages and cultures understand the importance of self-examination and thus helping in earlier diagnosis and reduction in mortality and morbidity of breast cancer. Women are encouraged to learn to examine their breasts regularly at specific times with the help of various methods, such as, artificial models, wall charts, pamphlets, magazines, videotapes, or slide but person to person teaching, if possible, especially a female health professional, is the most effective method. Self-examination of the breast is simple, safe, non-invasive, and inexpensive technique and can be practised more easily and effectively in a relaxed and comfortable place and time of her own. Some women may argue that the self-examination of the breast enhances the risk of unknown fear and anxiety for invasive procedures and expense, which may affect them either physically or psychologically or by both, but recent studies show the benefit out ways such argument. The best-informed professionals with whom the women feel relaxed, comfortable and confident should carry out the educational process. An adequate time should be devoted to the teaching process with emphasis on different changes in the normal situation, such as, with or without menstrual period, during a pregnancy and lactation period, and in abnormal condition. At first, by careful inspection followed by step by step palpation of the whole breast. A regular examination, if possible, once a month soon after the completion of menstrual period when the hormonic effect is negligible and thus resulting less chance of misleading results. The same regular monthly examination should also be carried-out during menopausal period.

The technique can be taught either at a doctor's surgery or in a special breast clinic, if possible, by a female doctor or by a well-trained nurse or a paramedic, or by a specialist physician, in the presence of an attendant. The examination room should be sufficiently and comfortably warm as well as the hands of the examiner. The woman should be asked to strip to the waist and there should be adequate provision for good lighting. The woman should be examined, in seated, in upright position, in leaning forward position and in supine position with slight elevation of the upper part of her body.

The inspection procedure (photograph no. 1-5) will be focussed on both the breasts first, then separately, with arms at the sides of the body, arms raised straight above the head, and then arms on the hips, pressing and relaxing, and finally bending forward from the waist. The ideas of these procedures are nothing but to increase the natural tension on the breast skin surface, so that any underlying condition can be brought to the surface for easy recognition.

On the breast, the woman should look from all possible angles first for any unusual asymmetry in sizes (normally the left breast is slightly larger than the right breast), or elevation of one breast. Second the shape — whether they are regular or irregular or distorted by any swelling. Third if there is any changes in the colour of the skin, any prominent veins — which show up more than normal, any nodules on the skin surface or any flattening or any dimpling or retraction or puckering of the normal breast contour. Any other changes on the breast skin surface, such as, naevi, warts, eczematous patch, ulcers must be noted because they might harbour some underlying pathology.

Thereafter, attention should be focussed on the nipple for any evidence of destruction, any retraction or inversion, any colour change, any deviation and displacement and any abnormal discharge with or without crusting including its character may signify some underlying pathology. Some discoveries of supernumerary nipple either single or multiple extending down the milk line on the chest, abdomen, and even to the vulva are not usual and should be noted.

Over the site of the areola, any cracks, fissure, swelling, ulcer, eczema, any abnormal discharge and diminution of the size of the areola limited either to the areola itself or as an extension process from the nipple also to be noted and reported accordingly. Very large areolas with prominent montgomery's tubercle and hair growths are not significant to any pathological condition other than psychological.

Finally, it is also important a heavy pendulous breast must be elevated manually to discover any pathological condition underneath.

Any retraction signs involving either breast skin surface, or nipple, or areola always represent destruction of tissue within the breast and signify presence of some underlying pathology.

After the completion of inspection procedure, the breasts should be palpated, one after another, with the flattened part of the finger pads (photograph no. 9) by pressing the breast tissue against the chest wall. The examination should cover the entire breast extending from the mid-sternal line to mid-axillary line and from the clavicle to one to two inches below the breast fold. A systematical but thorough examination of the whole breast either in a circle, clockwise or anticlockwise, strip wisely — from one side to the other or by individual quadrants (photograph no. 6-7-8-10-11-12-13-14) with particular attention to the axillary tail and area beneath the areola. A variable finger pressure is helpful in detecting and confirming deeper lesions, if any, but painful pressure should be avoided. The palpation is best carried out, especially in supine position after placing a small pillow under the scapula of the examining breast, first with an arm above the head with elbow bent and then down. Feeling especially the outer part and up towards the axila (axillary tail area, Photograph no. 15-16-17) should complete the examination. The examination of the breast in supine position is the most critical part of the entire process. The exact location for any masses, any tender areas, any thickening of the breast tissue and the character of the breast tissue in general as well as mobility of the breast whether fixed or freely mobile can only be detected by this way. The process should be repeated to the other side (photograph no. 18) routinely and a body lotion or talcum powder may be helpful for the smooth and uniform sliding motion over the breast surface. Depending on the size of the breasts, diagnostic accuracy can be achieved by giving sufficient time for examination, preferably three to five minutes for each breast, the method and the adequate experience of the learning process by the individual is a valuable tool for further investigations.

SELF EXAMINATION — PROCEDURE
(Look-Stretch-Lift-Press)

INSPECTION
(As in Photographs Number 1 to 5)

- Observe carefully and thoroughly sitting infront of a mirror from all possible angles — both the breasts first, then separately.

- Observe anything unusual — not either seen or noticed before — on the whole of the breast surface and then on the nipple and surrounding area.

- Lift heavy and enlarged breast by the hand and observe any changes underneath.

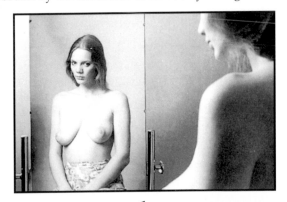

1

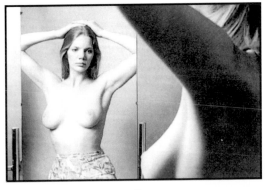

2

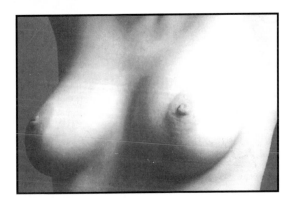

3

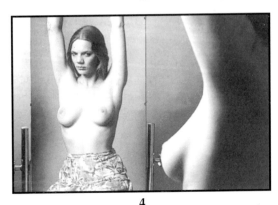

4

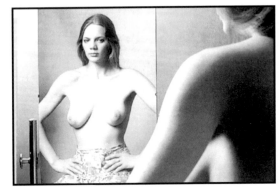

5

PALPATION
(As in photographs No. — 9, 6 to 8 & No. — 10 to 18)

- Use flattend part of the finger pads (as in photograph no-9) — palmer surface (innerside) of the hand.
- Palpate both the breasts, one after another, step by step right hand for the left breast and left hand for the right breast.
- Palpate whole breast either in circular way — clockwise or anticlockwise or by individual quadrants with special attention to the axillary area.
- Lie on a flat surface with your head on a small pillow. Slightly raise your left shoulder by placing a folded towel underneath it, and keep your left arm by your side (for left breast — photographs no — 6-7-8-10-11-12-13-14).
- Next raise your arm above your head with your elbow bent for easier examination of the outer part of the breast as well as the armpit — (photographs no — 15-16-17)
- Repeat the same examination procedure (reverse way) on the other side (photograph no-18).

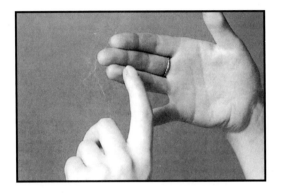

9

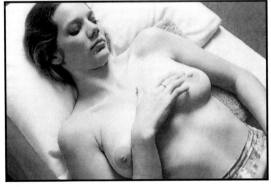

6

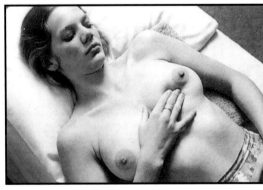

7

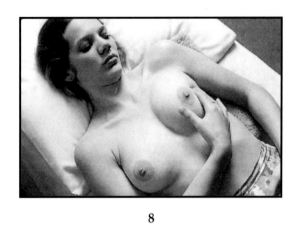

8

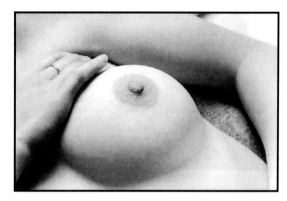

10

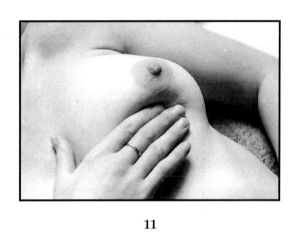

11

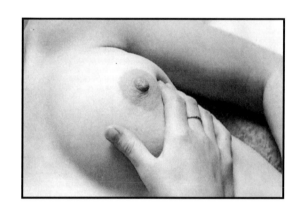

12

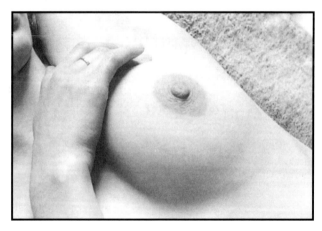

13

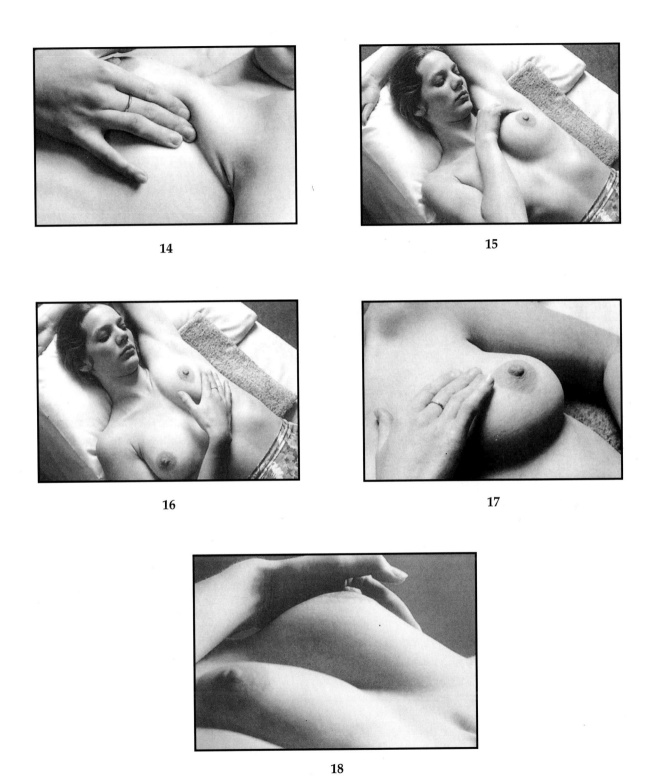

14

15

16

17

18

Remember—Regular breast self-examination may help to save your life.

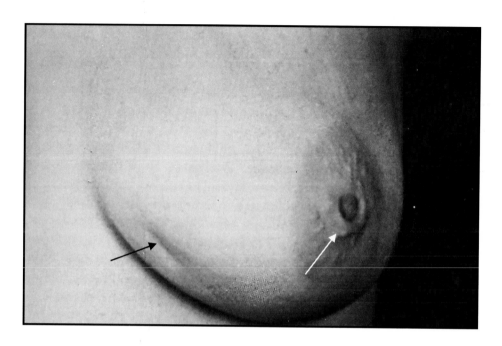

Changes in the breast contour—carcinoma of the left breast.
Showing dimpling of the skin in the lower and inner quadrant of the left breast.
Note: Retraction (inversion) of the nipple started.

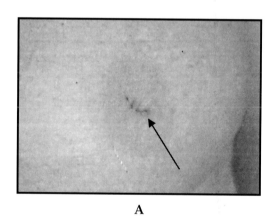

A

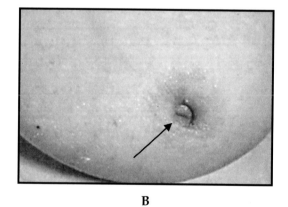

B

Nipple retraction due to (**A**) benign (duct ectasia) pathology and to (**B**) direct involvement with cancer.

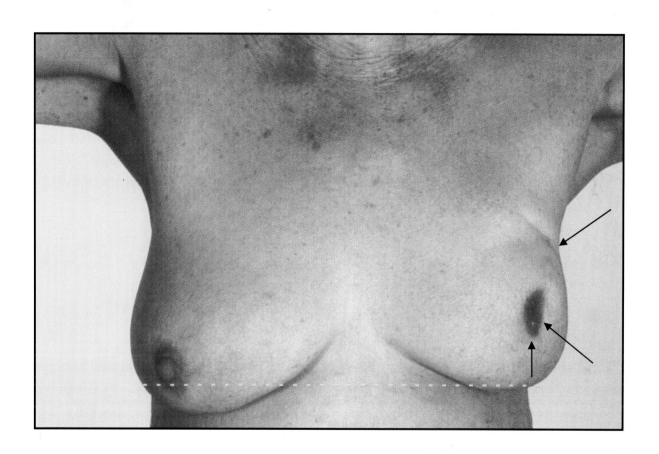

Carcinoma of the left breast showing dimpling of the skin, retraction of the nipple—lifted upwards and outwards.

CHAPTER 6

Breast -feeding and Problems

The key success of breast-feeding for a healthy, lively and contented baby depends on adequate advice, support and encouragement during pregnancy and puerperium. A mother who wishes to breast-feed her baby should be familiar with the technique before the delivery. Throughout generations much advice has been offered by doctors, midwives and family members on the best method of breast-feeding by way of practical demonstrations, as well as by illustrated literature and books, especially during her antenatal care period. After delivery, but before each feed a mother should assume a comfortable and relaxed position, whether sitting or lying, to feed her baby initially for a short period of two to three minutes, alternately on each breast. Feeding times are then gradually increased up to ten minutes or more on each side to satisfy the need of the baby. To promote a good supply of milk for nourishment and healthy growth of the baby great care must be taken to avoid mouth infection for the baby and the infection of the breast. At the same time the mother should also have a nutritious diet to provide a sufficient amount of milk for the baby.

Few would deny the value of breast-feeding, which is best, because -

- it provides essential nutritional, immunological and metabolic need for growth and development,

- it is easily available and ready for feeding the baby at any time and anywhere in the universe,

- it is the cheapest and best food for the baby and it helps to reduce the maternal blood loss during this period,

- it minimises the risk of pathogens and pollutants transmitted through breast milk but transmission of HIV viruses requires further research,

- it also controls the fertility by prolonging the amenorrhoeic phase and thus helping the mother to loose weight naturally,

- it creates neonatal maternal bonding by intimate and direct contact through somato-sensory stimulation, which may reduce the incidence of sudden infant death in certain communities. Lack of maternal bonding, as seen in western-style neonatal practices, separating the mother and the new-born, though controversial, may be linked with the development of psychological maladjustment in future life (for example - shyness, hyperactivity, violence or aggressiveness, etc.). Also, it has been noticed in artificial breast-feeding, there may be a greater risk of developing infections, such as, a gastrointestinal, necrotising enterocolitis, respiratory, urinary tract and ear etc,

- prolonged breast feeding from one breast per feed with equal emptying of both breasts at each feed for a long period, three months or more, although not a fool proof, may reduce the incidence of infant colic, better neurological development and breast engorgement. Recent studies suggests that by prolonging the breast-feeding time over a number of times may reduce the chance of developing breast and ovarian cancer, hip fractures and low bone density, childhood insulin-dependent diabetes mellitus and allergy (for examples — eczema, asthma and wheezing).

A further research work about the health benefits of breast-feeding to be continued particularly on the development of cardiovascular disease in later life, childhood cancer, cot death, rheumatoid arthritis, multiple sclerosis, acute appendicitis, tonsillectomy, dental health and obesity etc.

A mother may also face certain difficulties in breast-feeding as a result of problems, whether congenital or acquired, confined either to herself or to the baby or both. The commonest problem she may have to face -

- when the nipples are poorly developed,

- when breasts become congested and hard, knotty and painful,

- when there is a crack in the nipple, causing severe pain during the feed,

- when there is a breast abscess,

- when the baby is suffering from an infection, cerebral trauma, or some congenital heart lesion,

- when the baby is too weak to take the breast-feed or may tire before a sufficient amount of milk has taken, as in premature babies,

- when the baby is very small and there may be disproportion between the size of the nipple and the baby's mouth,

- when a baby may have congenital defects, such as, harelip, cleft palate, thus creating mechanical difficulty,

- when there is an over distended stomach of the baby with air causing discomfort thus refusing to take the breast,

A mother, under certain circumstances, should avoid breast-feeding when there is evidence of severe heart or kidney disease, puerperal mania — where the baby is at risk, and in active pulmonary tuberculosis.

A mother is more likely to continue to breast feed her baby if they have been breast-fed themselves, or breast-feed a previous child or watched a mother to breast-feed and also thought about the process and studied in a prenatal courses, and especially elderly woman in low socio-economic class group.

A mother is more likely to either end or does not wish to breast-feed her baby because of her -

- feelings about one's body and nudity, sexuality and pregnancy,

- early life experience and the quality and quantity of contact with her mother,

- relationship with the baby's biological father,

- developmental crises and geographical location,

- inadequate preparation during the antenatal period and insufficient milk,

- fear of loosing erotically arousing shape and thus reducing sexual pleasure.

A mother always should keep nipples clean, dry and soft after each feed with application of a bland cream or ointment (lanolin based). They should be cleaned and washed either with sterile water or lukewarm plain water before each feed to remove the cream. Sometimes airing the nipples is very important between the feeds. The use of local antiseptic cream or alcohol spirit swabs should be avoided, as these preparations are destructive to the nipples by making more dryers. Normally, the nursing mother may have to express her milk manually just before the feed to reduce the size of the swollen nipple and areola to accommodate the baby's mouth to avoid air sucking. Excessive and vigorous expression of the milk between the feed encourages continued engorgement and discomfort and therefore this practice should be avoided. Early treatment of soreness, cracks, and fissures, if any, in the nipple is very important. An excessive breast engorgement with milk some time requires urgent and immediate attention to reduce the pain and discomfort. If neglected, mastitis and later a breast abscess may follow.

The excess of milk can be removed by way of gentle massage or with the use of a breast pump machine. A well supported and good fitting brassiere pulls the breast upwards and inwards to reduce the discomfort and pain whereas an exceedingly tight brassiere restricts the blood supply to the breast and thus causing more harm than good. Icebags are particularly helpful during the engorgement period by way of reducing congestion and thus soothing cracked nipples. In extreme cases, mild analgesic tablets can be prescribed with caution.

If the mother is not going to breast-feed her baby, for any reason, lactation can be suppressed by a variety of methods, either by single or combined methods, such as, ice-bags, moderately tight and comfortable support of the breasts and analgesic tablets but not by hormone preparations. At the same time the mother should be taught how to feed her baby artificially.

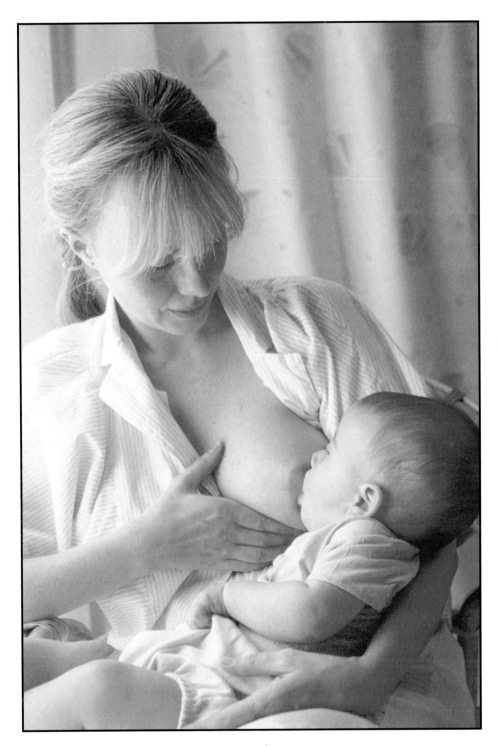

Breast-Feeding

Anatomical illustration and well catched nipple by the baby

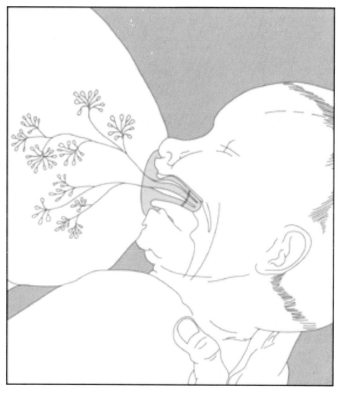

★ Good support at the baby's neck by the mother.

★ Ampulla well-within the baby's mouth.

★ Having uninterrupted good flow of milk.

★ Baby is close to the breast and less chance of air sucking.

★ Make sure baby's nose is not obstructed for breathing against the breast.

★ Both mother & baby must be in comfortable position - sitting or lying.

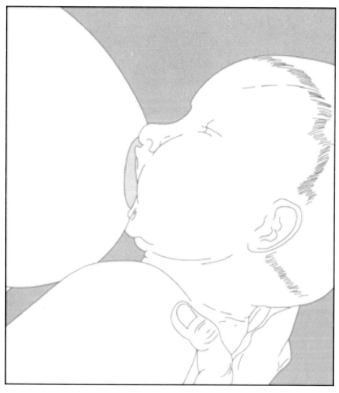

Anatomical illustration and not well-catched nipple by the baby

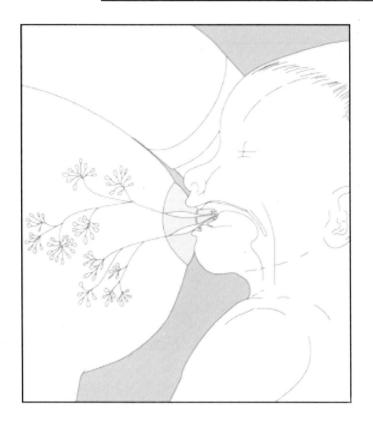

★ No support at the baby's neck by the mother.

★ Ampulla well-out side the baby's mouth.

★ Having poor flow of milk.

★ Baby is away from the breast and more chance of air sucking causing distended abdomen and colicky pain after the feed.

★ Baby may need too often feeding.

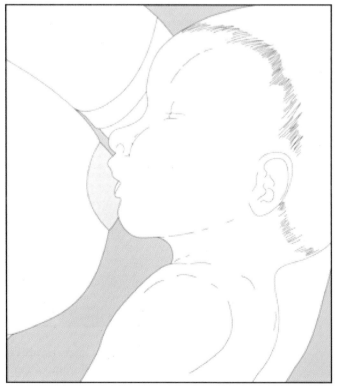

Lactational Mastitis

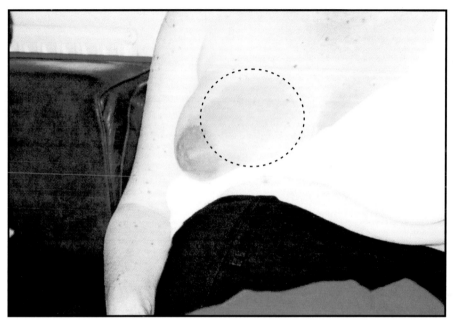

<u>Mother with mastitis</u>

The mother's breast-feeding technique was observed and suggestions for improvement were made

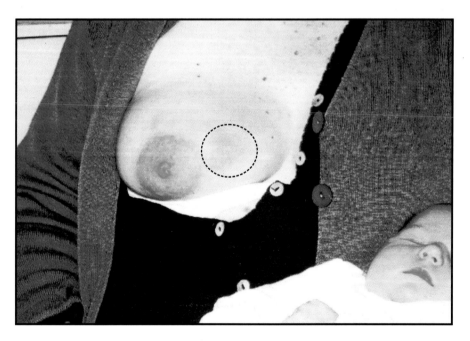

The same mother, two days later. Improved breast-feeding technique had resulted in more efficient milk removal and the mastitis resolved. The mother received no other treatment.

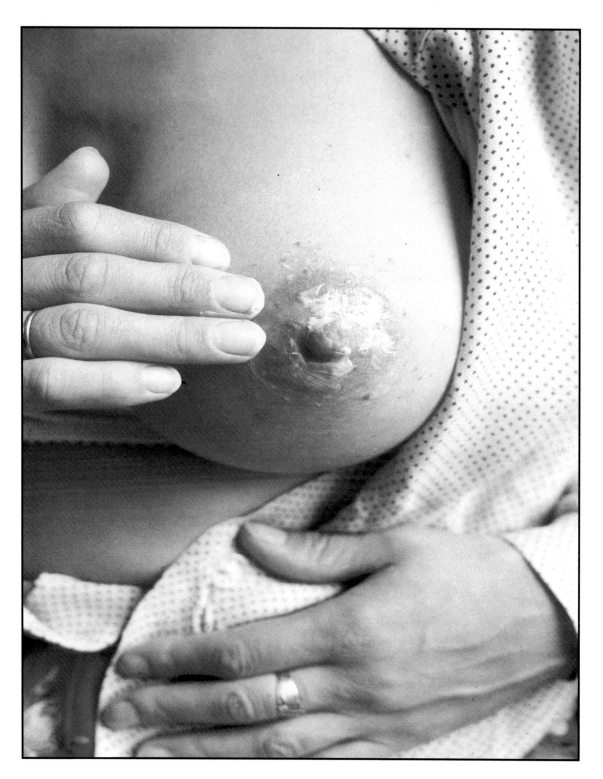

Local application of cream – nipple and surrounding areas

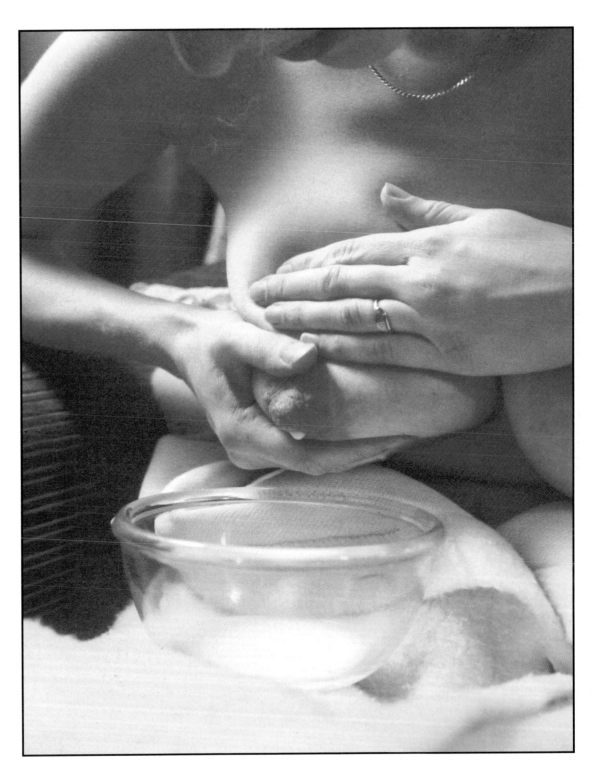

Milk expression from congested breast by hand.

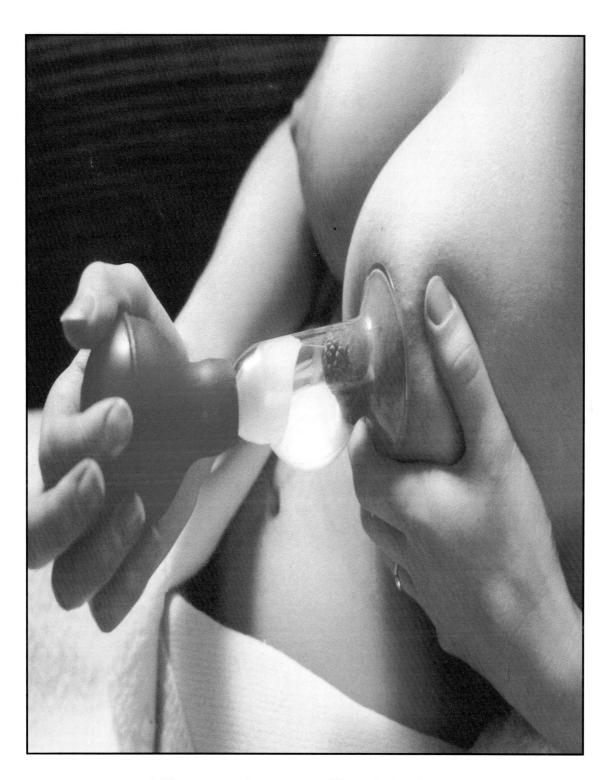

Milk expression from congested breast by hand pump.

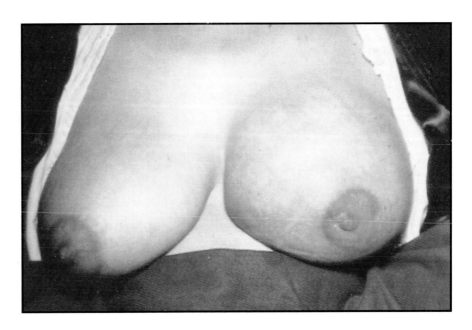

Non-lactating abscess of the left breast.

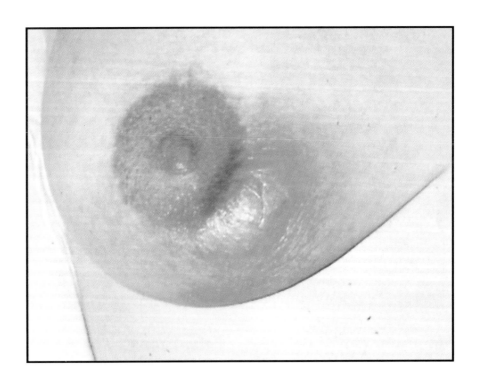

Non-lactating abscess of the right breast.

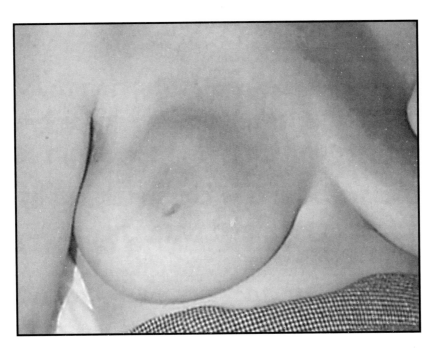

Peripheral breast abscess – (before treatment)

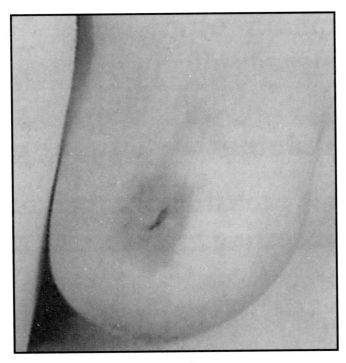

Peripheral breast abscess – (after treatment
by recurrent aspiration and oral antibiotics)

CHAPTER 7

Breast Nipple and Disorders

The nipples are conical protuberances at the tip of each breast and contain erectile tissue surrounded by pigmented area called the areola. Normally, they are usually at the same horizontal level and point outwards and downwards. The thick and corrugated skin of the nipple contains several invisible openings of the lactiferous ducts. Beneath the areola, areolar glands normally secrete an oily substance to keep the nipples supple and healthy.

Apart from normal character, particular attention to be focussed on any abnormality in the nipple, such as, presence of prominence or depression, any displacement in any direction, any abnormal discharge — with or without crusting including its nature, any fissures or cracks, any eczematous patches, or any ulceration. Presence of any single or multiple supernumerary nipples in the chest, abdomen, and even to the vulva should also be noted and reported accordingly.

Supernumerary Nipple :

These nipples are rarely seen in the milk line extending from axilla to groin on each side of the body but the most frequent site is in the axilla. They have been found to be active during the period of menstruation and lactation under the influence of hormones. They can be mistaken for a naevus.

Nipple Pain :

It is the commonest and most frequent complaint especially, by lactating mothers. It is mainly due to a failure to take necessary and proper care of the nipples immediately before and after delivery. A mother should take care of the nipples as early as possible in preparation for lactation to avoid future complications by regular washing, cleaning and keeping them soft and healthy, if necessary, with the help of a bland cream after each feed.

The incidence of painful, tender and traumatised nipples can be prevented or minimised significantly by appropriate nursing technique and positioning, either sitting or lying, by the lactating mother. At the first sign of any symptoms, if necessary, breast-feeding should be stopped on the affected side but the feeding to be continued on the less painful side with caution. To prevent a trauma to the nipple by a forceful suction by the baby for smooth milk flow, a gentle manual expression before starting any breast-feed will reduce such injury. The feeding frequency can be altered, either to keep the same regime or to be increased depending on the condition of the nipple. The suction pressure on the same part of the nipple as well as emptying of all the lobes of the breast can be minimised by rotation of the nursing position. The affected nipple can also benefit simply by exposure to fresh air between each feed. A proper elevation of the breasts with a firm but comfortable fitting nursing brassier with wide straps and nipple shields can greatly reduce the nipple pain. Sometimes, it is helpful to have a warm shower or bath before a feed. A mild analgesic and antibiotics, especially in severe cases, can be given with caution though a combination of analgesics and anti-inflammatory tablets can be prescribed under supervision only in special circumstances in an institution.

Nipple Retraction :

In this condition, the tip of the nipple lies below the level of the surrounding skin surface due to deficiency of the muscle tissue or flattening of the erectile tissue or by both. At puberty, the retraction of the nipple is a rare condition and may be due to developmental abnormality. Sometimes, retraction of the nipple may be possible as an after math of mastitis of infancy. Slight retraction of the nipple may be normal with some woman but a regular supervision will avoid future disaster.

Nipple retraction is the commonest cause of nipple asymmetry. The retraction of the nipple is usually caused by carcinomatous fibrosis not only within the tumour itself but also in the surrounding breast tissue. The fibrosis process may be either due to chronic inflammation or due to fat necrosis. The retraction is sometimes exaggerated with the application of mammography breast compression. A scar formation, secondary to some previous surgical procedures around the subareolar ducts causing them to thicken and shorten thus the nipple area becomes flattened and finally retracts.

Inversions of the nipple that can be corrected moderately easily by applying gentle manual pressure around the areola and should be differentiated from a retracted nipple. It is usually a long-standing process, often bilateral, which may occur in normal women. Thus, the diagnostic significance of the retraction of the nipple is very important and medical advice must be sought either in breast clinic or at doctors' surgery.

Nipple Eczema :

It is a rare condition, usually bilateral in origin and presenting eczematous features elsewhere in the body. A woman with this condition should be examined fully for a breast lump. A simple biopsy may be required in the absence of a lump, even if the eczema healed recently, to confirm the diagnosis.

Nipple Discharge :

Nipple discharge whether normal or abnormal is always a significant sign and may accompany several breasts' conditions. It may be unilateral or bilateral. Usually, local causes produce unilateral discharge whereas bilateral discharge is due to general and systemic causes. The nipple discharge may be caused by some tranquillisers, steroids, the oral contraceptive pill, and occasionally by digoxin and diuretic medication. The nipple discharge related either pregnancy or non-pregnant conditions, varied widely in amount, in appearance and in consistency, such as -

* **Witches' Milk:** is seen temporarily in a new-born baby in response to a maternal hormone for a short period of three to four weeks. It is yellowish in colour and affects both male and female infants,

- **Colostrum:** is normally seen in the early and later part of pregnancy due to increased blood supply to the breast as well as the hormonic effect. It is a thick yellowish fluid containing large fat globule, the colostrum corpuscles, high in minerals, low sugars, moderates in protein, antibiotics and with high calorific value,

- **Milk Secretion** (Physiological Lactation): it normally follows the colostrum secretion after delivery of the baby and this is maintained as long as the nursing stimulation continues. It is bluish-white in colour and contains mainly protein, fat, carbohydrate, vitamins and minerals,

- **Pale-white Discharge:** it either represents excess secretion by the lubricating cells or is a sign of mild chronic infection as seen in duct ectasis (dilatation of any tubular vessel). It commonly occurs in the perimenopausal as well as menopausal women due to primary dilatation of the major ducts. It is a benign condition but may signify an underlying carcinoma or a breast abscess,

- **Purulent Discharge:** it occurs in any infection and signifies a well-developed breast abscess,

- **Blood Stained Discharge:** it is normally seen in intra-ductal papilloma or in a duct carcinoma and needs urgent attention,

- **Black or Green Discharge:** this is either due to the altered colour of the blood from the ductal carcinoma or due to secondary retention cysts of fibroadenosis and women should consult their doctor for further investigation,

- **Pale-watery Discharge:** is a condition where there is flow of milk at intervals after cessation of a normal breast-feeding period. The amount of milk secretion lost each day varies a considerable amount and may be either spontaneous or associated with infertility, amenorrhoea, and ovulatory dysfunction. Normally the breasts are significantly flaccid, as in galactorrhoea, and there is no obvious external sign of great activity as found in pregnancy and puerperium.

Galactorrhoea :

In this condition there is an excessive flow of milk-like secretion due to various causes but the true incidence is unknown. It is a well-known condition for centuries and is often associated with a reproductive dysfunction. Many women with mild galactorrhoea do not seek any medical advice if there are no menstrual irregularities.

The most common cause of galactorrhoea is high normal or elevated prolactin level in the blood due to a prolactin-secreting tumour of the anterior pituitary gland. The presence of an extra-cellular tumour may also increase the prolactin level in the blood. Several physiological conditions, such as, sleep, exercise induced stress, sexual intercourse, breast stimulation either manually or by a breast pump other than in pregnancy and in breast-feeding, also increases the blood prolactin level. The other causes of hyperprolactinemia are often found in association with drugs, for example, phenothiazines, digitalis, reserpin, methyldopa, metoclopromide, marijuana, heroin and particularly with hormone therapy. Most women with normal menstrual function only seek advice from their doctors, if they are unduly worried. If this condition is reduced to one or two drops or stopped following temporary cessation of either drug's intake or physiological condition, as stated earlier, nothing more needs to be done other than reassurance.

Management of galactorrhoea depends on causes and should be supported by diagnostic evaluation. Drug related galactorrhoea has to be weighed-up against the merits before taking any further action. Reassurance and bromocriptin are now considered the treatment of choice for galactorrhoea.

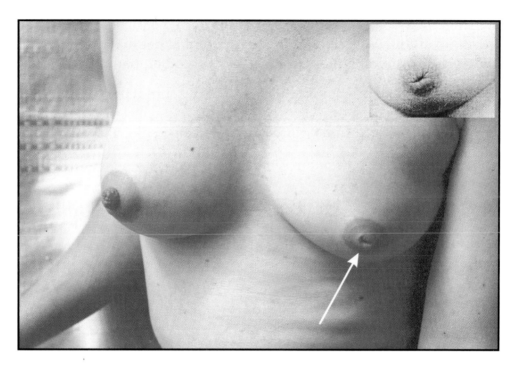

Retraction (inversion) of the left nipple.

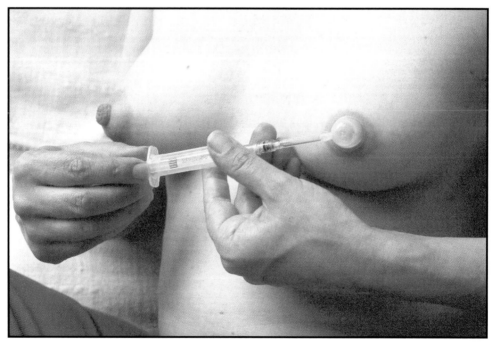

Retraction (inversion) of the left nipple – (correction procedure).

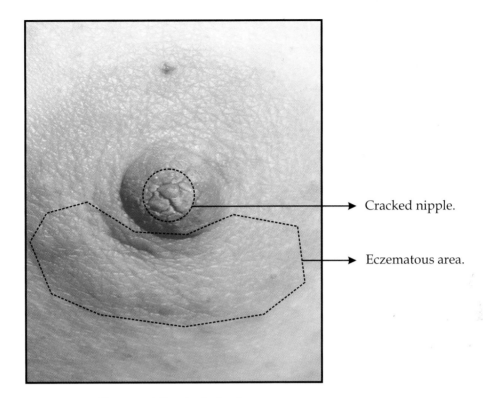

Cracked nipple.

Eczematous area.

Eczema / Cracked nipple.

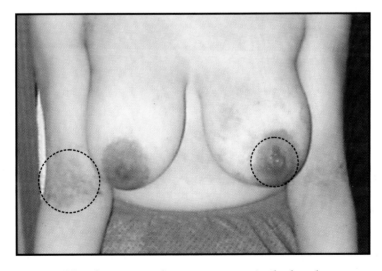

Nipple eczema also note eczema in the hand.

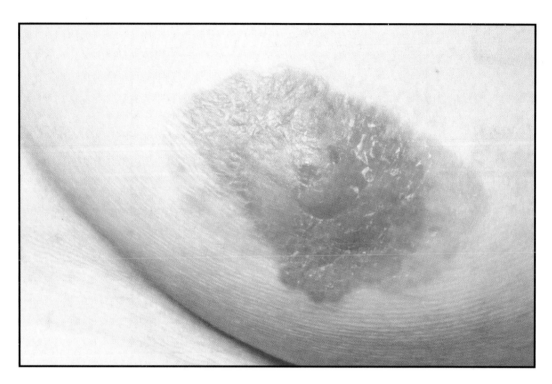

Paget's disease of the nipple.

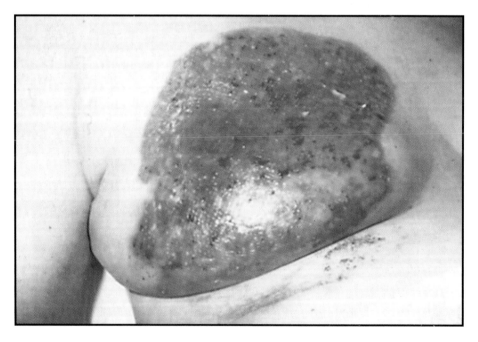

Paget's disease occupying a large area of the breast.

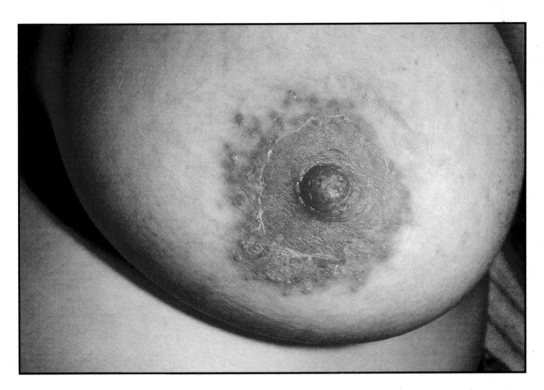

Candidiasis of the nipple and areolar area.

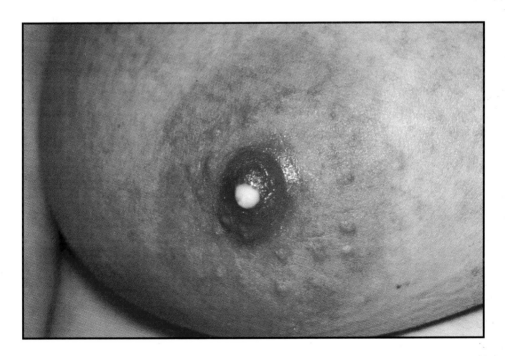

Galactorrhoea

CHAPTER 8

Breast Pain

Breast pain is a common presenting symptom and does not suggest any serious pathology. Cyclical breast pain occurs in almost 90 percent of women, as physiological, during their reproductive lifetime and should be differentiated from non-cyclical pain. Women under the age of 30 with breast pain, provided there is no indication of a malignancy and palpable discrete lump, need nothing other than reassurance. On the other hand, if the breast pain is occurring in the older postmenopausal group of women, a careful history, full clinical examination and a mammography will determine the exact cause of such concern. Normally the symptoms, such as, pain and tenderness, swelling, soreness, lumpiness, nodularity and even palpable thickening in the breasts are noticed, especially in the upper and outer quadrant, as they are hormone dependant. A simple explanation of the physiological nature of the breast pain and its relationship with the menstrual cycle, building up to a climax just before the period will be sufficient to allay anxiety. Normally, this type of breast pain subsides after the menopause but in persistent and severe cases whether in younger or older women, may adversely affect their life style (for example, exercise, swimming, sexual life, etc.). Careful assessment especially by family history, clinical examination as well as some form of breast imaging tests, such as, mammography or ultrasonography, will be mandatory. According to the severity of the breast pain, most women will benefit from wearing a good supporting brassiere, especially at night time or using some form of mild analgesic tablet or vitamin B-6. An oral contraceptive preparation either progesterone only pills or low dosages of combined pills for a short period of time may also relieve such breast pain. Treatment with bromocriptine, danazol, and tamoxifen, for a great minority of women should be tried for a short period of time under hospital specialists' supervision with full explanation of their benefits and side effects. Unexplained breast pain may be considered to be psychological in origin although recent studies of women with breast pain do not support this theory.

The other causes of breast pain may be found in mastitis, breast abscess, and rapid distension of a simple cyst and in peri-areolar duct ectasia — it is a chronic inflammatory process with a tender lump at the areolar edge. This may discharge through the skin causing mammary fistula.

Mastitis is an infectious process of the breast occurring most frequently during the lactation period or shortly thereafter. It may occur at any age, most often in primipara, during the first two to three weeks and sometimes as late as six months or more, after delivery. For most cases it is unilateral and more frequently institutional rather than domiciliary practice. Mastitis is characterised by a high temperature, localised erythema (a reddish patchy area), and lumpy, hot tender breast with continuous pain on the affected side. These signs may be associated with nausea, vomiting, malaise, and often flu-like symptoms, and palpable tender axillary glands.

Acute puerperal mastitis may be due to entry of some disease producing germs, commonly known staphylococcus, through a crack or abrasion on the nipple by way of one of the milk ducts.

At the outset of mastitis more than 50 percent of cases, a blood culture has repeatedly failed to reveal any convincing evidence of such infection. Normally, it begins in one lobe, but may extend to other areas. Apart from nipple trauma, maternal tiredness, poor nursing technique, marked reduction in breast care between the feeds, and poor milk flow during sucking may be the contributory factors of duct infection. Breast engorgement due to a stasis of the milk followed by clot formation in the ducts and in their tributaries form an excellent culture medium for the germ to grow rapidly and thus spread the infection. An early detection may help to avoid pus formation and thus prevent development of a breast abscess. In short, mastitis can be managed by bed rest, comfortable support with nursing brassiere, extra-fluid intakes, initiations of breast-feed on the unaffected side, regular emptying of the milk from the infected breast either by gentle manual expression or with a breast pump. In mild to moderate conditions an analgesic tablet, such as, paracetamol is sufficient to control the pain but in severe cases an antibiotic with or without non-steroidal anti-inflammatory drugs may be prescribed with caution and under proper supervision only. If neglected or delayed, it will rapidly develop to a breast abscess.

The breast abscess, has some characteristic features as in mastitis, and can be recognised by throbbing pain, oedema, and fluctuant area in the centre. It usually occurs in the upper and outer quadrant of the breast. The management of the breast abscess is similar to mastitis and in confirmed cases, a total stoppage of breast-feeding to the affected breast and surgical drainage is the choice of treatment. To avoid increased blood loss, risk of fistula and risk of ductal occlusion; a great care must be taken, during the surgical procedure. A supra-mammary abscess occurs as a result of suppuration of the superficial lobule of the breast or sebaceous gland.

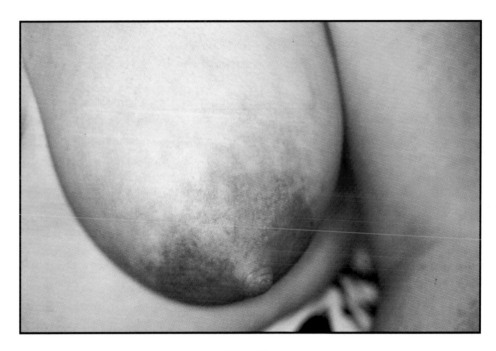

Mastitis

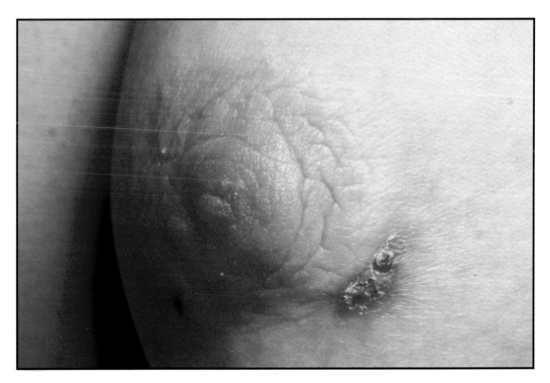

Fistula of the Breast

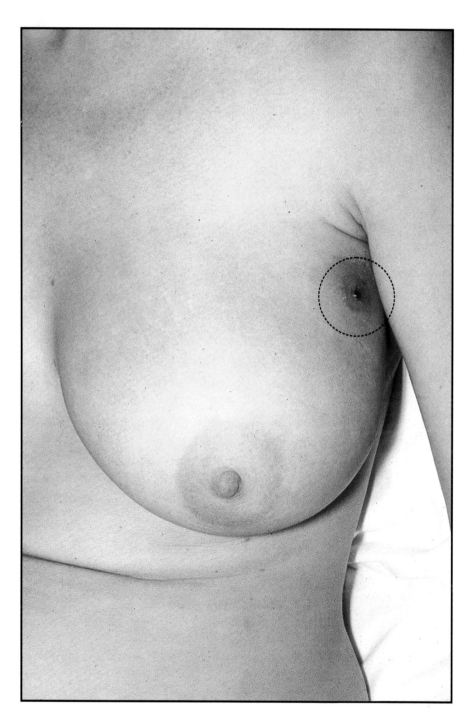

Breast abscess

CHAPTER 9

Breast Screening

The main aim of breast screening is to detect the breast cancer when it is in its early stages and before it has had the chance to spread to the surrounding structures. The death rate from the breast cancer, in women between 40 and 50, is the highest in Britain (one in 12) than anywhere else in the world. Although, the incidence rate of breast cancer is not high in this country but the survival rates are poor because of various reasons. The disease may be more aggressive in Britain, the patchy services and poor treatment of the disease (any delay between the women noting an abnormality and receiving definite treatment). Many areas have no specialist's unit other than general hospital and general surgeon with limited experience in breast surgery, and shockingly sometimes longer waiting times to see a specialist breast surgeon.

At present, under the National Breast Screening Programme, women between 50 and 70 years of age are invited for routine mammograms in every three years. Women aged 65 and 70 or over in certain age limit areas, are only given mammograms on request. Several studies have shown that by routine screening of women over 50, it is more effective in reducing mortality and morbidity than in younger women under 35.

Very few women get breast cancer in their teens and in early 20's but routine screening under 50 can, do harm than good. First, there is marked density in the breast in younger women, which makes it difficult to diagnose breast cancer accurately. This may increase false positive results, which may lead to unnecessary surgery. Second, some women may be referred for surgery for border line tumours which would have regressed anyway and third, some women may have to attend 30 years of breast screening clinic with no increase in protection value other than psychological trauma and unnecessary radiation exposure. Pregnant women should not have mammograms because of the radiation effect on the baby.

Latest clinical evidence suggested by some cancer specialists show a further reduction in death from breast cancer can be achieved by extending this service to all women up to the age of 70 years without any age limit restriction. But others believe such benefit to be balanced against the increasing cost, increased work load, unnecessary anxiety, and are not certain whether older women would come forward or not.

A special breast unit should work like a team and consist of a breast surgeon, experienced radiologist and well-trained radiographer, histopathologist, an oncologist (a cancer drug therapy specialist), breast cares nurse, chemotherapy experienced nurse, physiotherapists and psychologists. Also, there should be an additional day care surgery facilities to carry out biopsy procedures, plastic surgeon for reconstruction of the breast following a surgery, if necessary, the provision of prosthesis department and social care group etc. If any government wants to reduce the death rate from breast cancer an adequate and proper investment must be made to provide such care all over the country in a proper manner.

In the past, various methods, such as, radioisotope studies, ductography, nipple cytology, trance-illumination light screening, and magnetic resonance imaging, etc. were used for breast screening or diagnosis of the breast cancer without any documented overall benefits other than expense. To date, apart from clinical examination, either by the women (breast self-examination), or by the general medical practitioner at the surgery, or by the breast specialist surgeon at the clinic, which is the commonest diagnostic aid in association with other methods, such as, mammography, sometimes ultrasonography and thermography. But the mammography is the commonest and is routinely performed for accurate and definite diagnosis of the breast cancer.

To evaluate cost-effectiveness of the programme, and to reduce the significant numbers of mortality and morbidity, the risk group should be invited and their personal details to be maintained properly. The women should be encouraged to attend this screening clinic by their general practitioners, the media, such as, a television and radio discussion programme, newspapers, and magazines, video tapes, and by posters, etc. by their own family and friends and to teach themselves the technique of breast self-examination. Also, high standards of the screening programme should be maintained by continuous improvement in the specialist programme, research, and treatment. A regular audit and review of both individual and breast screening programme results are essential to achieve a set target.

Mammography :

It is an X-ray examination of the breast, and is one of the commonest and valuable diagnostic tools available for routine breast screening procedures all over the world. Over the years, advances in technology, by improving image quality and a dramatic reduction in radiation, mammography alone detects nearly 85 to 90 percent of all breast cancers before a physician or if a woman feels a lump. It should be performed at any age when clinical findings lead a physician to suspect cancer. The breasts in adolescent women are primarily consisted of fibroglandular tissue and only a small amount of radio-lucent fat. With advancing age, the glandular tissue atrophies to fatty tissues and the connective sheathes, and becomes visible on mammograms more easily.

Thus, the breasts of older women are mainly consisted of radio-lucent fat and this helps to detect the cancers even it is only a few millimetres in sizes. The procedure and the positions of the women vary with the type of machine in use for this examination. The breast may be gently compressed between two plates, or may be laid on the top of a flat surface or allowed to hang down or sucked into a cavity. The procedure is usually painless and takes about 20 to 30 minutes, although some women feel notably uncomfortable. Mammographic examination should consist of at least two views of each breast. A medio-lateral oblique view shows the maximum amount of breast tissue including deeper structures in the upper and outer quadrant and in the axillary tail. A direct lateral view with a craniocaudal view usually determines the exact location of a nonpalpable breast lesion. The breast compression method improves resolution by preventing breast movement, decreases a radiation dose by reducing the breast thickness, separates overlying structures and also differentiates the cystic and solid masses. An additional view may be performed when an abnormality suggestive of cancer is identified. Mammography is expensive and always needs special film and processing methods as well as highly trained technicians and radiologists to interpret the films. The frequency of mammography varies depending on analysis of individual risk factors but the best frequency is probably between 18 months and two years. The commonest risk factors are family history — mother, sister, and daughter, onsets of menstrual period before the age of 12, have not had any children, had a late onset of a menopause, and have used hormone replacement therapy for longer than ten years after the age of 50. Cancer risk from mammographic examination is very small compared with an incidence of breast cancer in general.

As various studies suggest mammography is the most effective aid for early detection of breast cancers even though properly performed mammograms failed to identify ten to 15 percent of breasts' cancers. Thus, some false negative mammograms may adversely affect the prognosis by delaying the biopsy and further treatment. The major reason for a false negative result is due to dense parenchymal tissue although radiographic techniques and errors in interpretation can be blamed. An abnormal mammography report does not need any further action other than reassurance by the general practitioner or by the clinic. Women with suspected or a proven tumour requires urgent appointment to see a cancer specialist at the clinic.

Ultrasonography :

In this method of examination, a high frequency sound waves are projected through the breast to create echoes between tissues of different density and then these return to the source and the reflections are detected and turned into images.

The most important clinical use of breast sonography is to differentiate between cysts and nonpalpable solid masses detected by mammography. The breast sonography also plays an important role in the evaluation and follow-up of patients with multiple cysts and in palpable masses and in suspected breast abnormalities, mainly associated with dense parenchymal tissue, which limits mammographic evaluation.

The breast sonography can be carried-out adequately either with an automated whole breast unit or a high frequency handheld unit. In breast cancer screening examinations, automated whole breast scanners are more valuable than handheld units because they produce sequential thin sections of whole breast images and are more accurate in localising the abnormalities. But the automated units are costly, need more space, and especially trained technologists, and take longer to a set-up. The handheld units are less expensive, and moderately quick and easy to operate. The handheld unit can also be used for needle-guided biopsy procedures. The intensity and frequency used in ultrasonography examination are completely harmless and so far no recorded fatality.

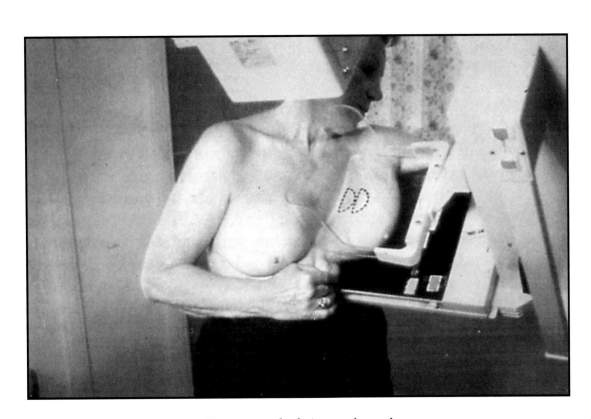

Mammography being performed.

CHAPTER 10

Breast Lump

Most women do not wish to divulge or discuss symptoms or any abnormality to their breasts because of the potential significance of their symptoms. Most of them feel ashamed to talk about as it is a personal matter, unimportant and time wasting. But these old trends are changing rapidly due to publicity through the media as well as, in particular, self-awareness of their wellbeing. To days women are more open and free to discuss any personal problems not only with the professionals but also with their friends and family and even take part in open discussion in the media, such as, in radios and in televisions.

Most women who consult their doctors with breast problems, such as, painful breast, breast lump, nipple discharge or retraction or deviation or skin changes or just feeling her breasts are not right, etc. show some sign of anxiety on their face. The age, menstrual status, accurate accounts of the symptoms, as well as full clinical examination, etc. are indicators either for referral or reassessment or reassurance. The average general practitioner probably sees about 20 cases of breast cancer in his or her lifetime and some of them may not feel confident about making a diagnosis. If there is any worry about the diagnosis at the back of doctors' mind not only the clinical and psychological grounds but also the medico-legal ground warrants her referral to the hospital for opinion and advice.

The aim of clinical examination is to detect any palpable abnormalities in the breasts and in the regional lymph nodes and should be performed routinely either at the doctor's surgery or at the breast clinic. The room should be comfortably warm as well as the flat surface of the doctor's hand. Then the women should be asked to undress to the waist and there must be provision of good lighting facility for thorough inspection and palpation.

During inspection, first the shape of the breasts, any asymmetry of the breasts and their movement, any sign of inflammation on the skin surface, any atrophy or colour change, any ulceration, etc. should be looked for. Second a special attention to be focussed to the nipples for any change of position, any local retraction or protrusion, evidence of any discharge and its nature or any duplication or any eczematous condition including any abnormal sign over the supraclavicular area, should be noted. The whole of inspection and the palpation procedures must be made in the presence of an attendant.

The breast should be observed with the women in sitting position facing the doctor initially, her arms resting at her sides, then slowly raised straight behind the head. Next, the women should be asked to put her hands on her hips and press, followed by bending forward position. Finally, the breasts should be observed while the woman is lying on her back at a 45-degree angle position.

Any abnormality noted during the inspection procedures should be confirmed by palpation. It is very important to find the texture of the normal breast first before examining the abnormal breast because it varies from woman to woman. In some women the breast texture is soft and smooth whereas in others it is firm, fibrous and glandular. To start with, opposite breast should be palpated with the palmer surface of the fingers, (i.e. with the hand flat) while the woman is lying down position with her arms at her sides. The breast should be palpated systematically by a gentle circular movement covering centre, four quadrants as well as axillary tail. Any firmness of the tissue or resistance to movement indicates more careful attention to the site in relation to the skin and deeper structures, whether fixed or not, its shape, size, surface edge, surface temperature, any tenderness and the consistency — solid or cystic. Finally, supraclavicular area and the axilla (armpit) should be palpated. The axilla can be examined either in sitting or standing position first with the woman's hand resting on the doctor's shoulder and secondly by allowing her arms to drop inwards towards the chest wall. These manoeuvres allow the chest muscles (pectoral muscles) to relax, so that the entire axilla can be examined thoroughly including the uppermost area. Any mild or gentle pressure causing pain or presence of any palpable lymph node and their size, shape, consistency and their relation with surrounding tissue; should be noted accordingly. The whole procedures should be repeated on the other side.

After carrying out full thorough examination, the doctor should try to make a definite decision whether there is a lump or any abnormality present, which is not always easy. If a lump or an abnormality cannot be detected, it is better to ask the woman to place her fingertip on the exact location where she thinks to be appropriate. If the woman can locates the precise spot without any hesitation, a further careful examination of the site should be made. If on the other hand, the woman is vague and picking no tissues between the fingers and moving her fingers in a different manner then she has no lump.

Now, the outcome of the examination is likely to be first. The woman has no lump and no other abnormality in the breasts. These are mainly young women and should be reassured with explanation as their symptoms and are advised to report back after one or two menstrual periods. These symptoms may be related to either some form of an injury or menstrual cycle. There is no need for immediate hospital referral but they should be encouraged to examine regularly their breasts (as explained in self-examination). Breast cancer under 25 is extremely rare. Second, the woman could have a lumpy breast but no true lump. This is the commonest symptom in women those who are in their 30's and early 40's. This may be bilateral with vague thickenings in the breast. This group of women should be re-examined at some different phases of their menstrual cycle, preferably, after the period to confirm their symptoms. If it is negative, the woman should be reassured and to be advised accordingly, whereas any uncertainty at the second visit (for example, persistence of lumpiness or abnormality) requires referral to the hospital is the safest and best way to reduce women's anxiety and correct diagnosis. A full discussion and explanation of the diagnosis will increase her confidence too. Third the woman has a definite lump. These groups are usually needed early, if not immediate, hospital referral for further investigations.

The nipple discharge, only blood stained and black or greenish type of discharge signifies underlying pathology and needs urgent attention.

Most of the women with breast abnormalities complain of change either in the breast size or in the nipple or a lump with or without pain and tenderness. Most breast lumps are benign and due to either breast inflammation, or a breast cyst or a non-malignant breast tumour.

Fibroadenomas :

These are the most common benign tumours encountered in all groups but particularly between menarche and 30 years of age. Being oestrogen dependent, they grow rapidly during adolescence and pregnancy up to the size of ten to 12 centimetres in diameter and regress after a menopause. The large size is not an indication of malignancy. They usually present a solitary, a freely mobile, lobulated, well-defined smooth surfaced tumour with a rubbery firm consistency and in various sizes, usually one to three centimetres in diameter. They are surrounded by fibrous capsule and the cut surface of the tumours shows pink or tan-white in colour. They are a solid and usually a nontender tumour, occur in any part of the breast. Malignant changes are rarely seen in fibroadenomas. They are usually diagnosed clinically and confirmed by imaging, ultrasound method for premenopausal groups or by mammography for postmenopausal groups.

Most young women can be treated conservatively and to be followed up every six months whereas others prefer to have a removal of the fibroadenomas either under local or general anaesthesia depending on the size, even only after the clinical diagnosis. In women aged over 40, excision is the best policy to ensure that the breast cancers are not missed.

Cysts :

Most cysts occur in the late reproductive years as the woman is approaching a menopause, but the commonest age groups are 30 to 50. Cysts are found in various sizes either in clusters or as a single cyst. Generally, they feel smooth and mobile and have a firm consistency due to distension. Larger cysts form fluctuant lesions, and usually contain brown colour fluid due to haemorrhage. A simple cyst usually disappears with aspiration and contains clear serous or straw-coloured fluid. In younger women the cysts are readily diagnosed by ultrasonography although a characteristic halo is the hallmark on the mammograms for menopausal women. The cystic fluid may be examined cytologically but it is unhelpful. Since there is no residual lump immediately either after the aspiration or at a follow-up, four to six weeks intervals at a different stage of a menstrual cycle, the woman can be discharged from the clinic with reassurance. If the fluid on aspiration is bloodstained or if it recollects or if there is no fluid on aspiration because of solidity of character of the cyst, the woman should be referred urgently for specialists' opinion.

Breast cytology plays an important role in the diagnosis of benign breast disease and requires an especially skilled team to collect samples and to interpret the smears by histopathologist. It is not a job for amateurs. The procedure usually is carried out under local anaesthesia.

A carcinomatous breast lump, often start as a painless lump, can grow anywhere in the breast — commonly in the upper and outer quadrant. An enlarging lump may distort the shape and size of the breast as well as the nipple. They are usually solid and in a late stage become fixed to the surrounding structures and manifested with pain, ulceration of the breast skin surface and sometimes the nipple. They also affect lymph nodes in the axillary and clavicular area and finally spread to the other parts of the body structures — liver, lungs, bone and brain etc.

CHAPTER 11

Breast Cancer and Causes

The exact cause of breast cancer is unknown. It is the single commonest cause of death affecting about one in 12 woman in Britain between 40 and 50 years of age. Till to date, hundreds of studies of all kinds, both nationally and internationally been done in the prevention of breast cancer but so far little has been achieved. Also major technical advances in diagnosis and intensive efforts to improve treatment quality has not been able to reduce the mortality and morbidity rate from breast cancer. Breast cancer is mainly hormonal and being multifactorial in origin, reflects interactions of many mechanisms. Two major risk factors have been identified — 'sex and age'. Breast cancer affects females almost entirely and increases with age.

Age :

The incidence of breast cancer related to age varies from countries to countries — higher in western countries than in Far Eastern countries. The incidence of breast cancer is low in women under 30 and with age it increases sharply between 40 and 50. The highest incidences usually have seen between the age group 60 to 70 and significantly drops after 80.

Hormonal and Reproductive Factors :

It has been known by large epidemiological studies that women who start menstruating early (before the age of 11) in life and who have a late onset of a menopause (after the age of 55 or more) have an increased risk of developing breast cancer. The cycles become longer, anovulatory and irregular in women with a late menopause and thus increase the level of unopposed oestrogen stimulation for longer periods. In other words, women with more regular menstrual cycles in life are at greater risk of developing breast cancer for the same reason.

An early menopause either due to bilateral salpingo-oophorectomy (removal of both ovaries and tubes) before the age of 35 or natural menopause before the age of 45 reduces the risk of developing breast cancer for less than half in women who have a natural menopause at age 55 or greater. Removal of one ovary is less protective than two ovaries and a hysterectomy (removal of the uterus) alone do not change the risk.

Women who have their first full term delivery after the age of 30 or older, and nulliparity, both increase the risks of developing breast cancer is about twice than those delivering their first child before 20 years of age. Women at highest risks are those who have their first child after 35. There may be a possibility of increased cancer risk, if the first pregnancy is interrupted during the first three months of pregnancy. Incomplete pregnancy, abortion after completion of the first full term pregnancy, increasing number of births, if they occur at an early age, may have little or no protective effect.

Family History :

The risk of developing breast cancer in a woman is two or more times greater if she had a family history of breast cancer, especially — a mother, sister or daughter (called first degree family relation) who developed the disease before the age of 50. Also women with first degree relatives with premenopausal bilateral breast diseases have a nine to a 14-fold increase in risk as compared with relatives with unilateral postmenopausal disease.

Breast cancers due to genetic mutations are often found in a small number of cases. It is not yet known how many abnormal genes are there to cause breast cancer. Recently, in families with genetic susceptibility, such abnormal genes called 'BRAC 1' and 'BRAC 2' is identified and there is only a 50 percent chance that this abnormal gene will be passed on to several family members through either sex. However, women who inherit this fault gene have a greater risk of developing breast cancer depending on age and family history. The incidences of increase are 12 percent by the age of 35, 50 percent by the age of 50, and 80 percent by the age of 80. Breast cancers with family history there are three fold increases with mother, sister, or aunt and a 14-fold increase with both mother and sister. Protection from developing breast cancer, for women who know they carry the faulty gene in advance, opt to have their breasts surgically removed before the disease shows-up. In families with genetic susceptibility to breast cancer there may also be other associated cancers, such as, cancer of the ovary, endometrium (linings inside the uterus) and colons. If a woman is unaffected by breast cancer at 65, despite strong family history of an early onset, probably she has not inherited the genetic mutation. Genetic screening is available under National Health Service on a limited basis.

Socio-economic Status / Lifestyle :

Breast cancer rates for the highest socio-economic class is 50 percent greater than that for the lowest. The difference is due to lifestyle factors in career-orientated women, having children in later and most likely do not wish to breast-feed their babies, amount of an alcohol consumption, and high standard of diet.

Recently, not only in Britain but also in other parts of the world, much of the attention and study has been focussed on diet and their relation in the development of the breast cancer. Some researchers believe that adopting healthy lifestyle, as for cardiovascular disease can reduce the risk of developing breast cancer. To achieve this, a diet containing excessive fat and meat consumption to be replaced with a low-fat, high fibre diet, fresh fruits and vegetables (if possible organic in origin) nuts, vitamin C and E, pulses, soya and cereal products, oily fish, an olive oil and garlic etc. It had been known that the body weight depends on a caloric intake. The influence of body weight affecting breast cancer risk varies in relation to a menopause. Some studies have reported that body weight (obesity) significantly increases the risk of developing breast cancer in postmenopausal women (two fold increases) than in premenopausal women.

There is conflicting opinion amongst experts, between alcohol consumption and the incidence of breast cancer, even though the risk is small, young women may increase their risk with moderate drink, say two to three units of alcohol per day, in association with other identified risk factors. Previously, it was thought that smoking has got little or no effect in the development of breast cancer. Recently, a new study suggests that there is an increased risk of developing breast cancer in women who started smoking in their teens. Childless women who smoked 20 or more cigarettes per day over a period of 20 years are likely to develop seven times more breast cancer than non-smokers.

Recent epidemiological studies involving 30 countries, shows' women are less likely to develop breast cancers are those who breast-feed their babies over a longer period for several times.

Radiation :

Exposure to radiation increases the risk of breast cancer and varies by age at exposure and may be strongest in childhood during the breast developmental stages. The incidence, thereafter, gradually falls with advancing age and becomes negligible over age 40 to 50. The incidence of breast cancer from modern X-rays and mammography is very little because it emits very small doses of radiation. But when an individual is exposed to atomic bomb radiation, the effect seems to be greater than expected, as evidenced in Japanese women, and particularly in association with other risk factors including family history and benign breast disease.

Benign Breast Disease :

Women who had a breast biopsy or who had a history of fibrocystic diseases have a two to four times the risk of developing breast cancer. Depending on tissue histology (for example - epithelial hyperplasia), which varies with menopausal status and a family history of breast cancer have increased risk of developing breast cancer up to six times a greater than of those without such condition.

Other Factors :

Reserpine, a hair-dyes, caffeine intake, worry, anger, death, divorce, stress, women of Jewish faith, living in urban areas rather than rural areas etc., may have some relation in the development of breast cancer. Women who worked in the pharmaceutical and agricultural industries and those live near hazardous waste sites and under power cables, VDU's operators etc., have been found to have some form of links, although debatable singly, with the development of breast cancer together with other major factors.

CHAPTER 12

Breast Cancer Management

Breast cancer is now widely accepted as a systemic disease and most of the women will not be cured even with the most extensive local treatments available today. To prolong life expectancy and to improve the quality of life, there has been a shift in the management of breast cancer, such as, participation of the patient in the treatment planning, improved surgical technique to provide confidence and self-image, and technological improvement in the diagnostic procedures, etc. The treatment varies from hospital to hospital and individual to individual depending on the stage of the disease and the age of the woman. The multi disciplinary team, depending on individual nature and extent of the tumour affected in a woman usually takes the treatment decisions. At the same time woman should have a full discussion and assessment before obtaining any consent for treatment. First, there must be a provision of full information about the types of treatment available to her (for example - surgery including breast reconstruction where applicable, radiotherapy and chemotherapy and hormone therapy), its aim, benefits and potential side effects. Second, a sufficient and reasonable time to be given to think and discuss with her family and partner, if any, and to consider treatment options available to her. Third, she should be given chance to meet breast cancer sufferers for advising and support. Finally, she should also expect information on follow-up services (for example - a prosthetic breast fitting department, psychological support and social support etc.), and thus reducing the complication afterwards.

Breast cancer treatment is becoming increasingly sophisticated and practice either in local or in systemic form, although, most women will have the treatment in the combination form. The local treatment consists of surgery and radiotherapy, to control local disease whereas the systemic treatment consists of hormonal manipulation and chemotherapy for advanced disease with the aim of inducing remission rather than cure.

Breast cancer is classified either in non-invasive (in situ) form or in invasive form. In non-invasive form cancer cells remain within the basement membrane of the terminal duct and lobular unit whereas in invasive form, the cancer cells spread outside the basement membrane of the ducts and lobules into the surrounding normal breast tissue, may even spread to lymph glands. In extreme cases, it spreads to other part of the body, such as, liver, bone and in the brain.

By Surgery :

The aim of surgical procedure in the management of breast cancer is -

- to secure long term control of the disease, local as well as regional lymph nodal areas, so that recurrence and distance spread can be avoided or delayed.

- to conserve the breast and their function as much as possible with a minimal deformity.

- to improve the quality of their life and their life expectancy.

Over the years, the knowledge of breast cancer biology and natural history and improvement in all aspects related to surgery including selection of a woman, made possible present day practice — a conservative surgical approach rather than previously used more mutilating radical approach.

Conservative breast surgery consists of either removal of the tumour (a primary site) with local excision (called lumpectomy) including one to two centimetres adjacent normal healthy breast tissue or a more extensive excision of the tumour with the involved quadrant of the breast (called quadrantectomy) including overlying skin. The greater the area of excision, the lesser the chance of recurrence of an incidence but the worse the cosmetic result, although the conservative approach appeals to many women.

The breast conservative surgery is suitable for women with a single clinical and mammographic lesion, tumour size less than four centimetres in diameter, neither too central nor too peripheral within the breast and if there is no clinical sign of a metastasis or nodal involvement.

Women with widely separated tumours in the same breast, mammograms reveals diffuse disease in many quadrants, relatively small breast, an elderly woman and ulcerated lesion are suitable for radical approach rather than either lumpectomy or quadrantectomy.

In some women, if there is any inaccuracy in clinical assessment at the time of operation, where a microscopic spread may have already extended beyond the visible margins of the primary tumour, that a surgical sampling of the regional node is important for future treatment. If the histology shows, deposit of cancer cells in the node radiotherapy should be given to the remaining breast and scrupulous clinical follow-up to be maintained. The negative results only need a scrupulous follow-up approach.

The total simple mastectomy operation, as far as the woman is concerned, is a radical procedure and about third of the women with localised breast cancers are not suitable for conservative surgery can be treated by this method.

In a total mastectomy, the entire breast including the nipple areolar complex is removed with preservation of the chest wall muscles whereas in a conventional radical mastectomy includes removal of the involved breast, the underlying pectoralis muscle and the axillary contents. The most common practice breast surgery is the total mastectomy with a limited axillary dissection or a surgical sampling of few nodes (known as simple mastectomy) is essential because it provides guidance to the prognosis and dictates additional methods of treatment, if required, later. By a simple mastectomy the primary site and adequate regional control can be achieved, while others prefer a simple mastectomy associated with full axillary nodal clearance (known as modified radical mastectomy) to avoid an unacceptable rate of a relapse. The success rate appears to be similar in both cases provided the selection of women and the stage of the disease were assessed thoroughly before the respective procedure.

Following a mastectomy operation various complications may be seen in varying proportion such as —

- bruising, swelling, and delayed healing,

- infection — is more common in older women, usually secondary to flap necrosis and treatment with prolonged catheter drainage. Rarely skin graft is necessary in areas of necrotic skin and appropriate antibiotic, if necessary, will resolve the problem,

- skin necrosis — in some women with poorly vascularised very thin skin may show discrete areas of skin necrosis as a result of axillary dissection,

- seroma — which is very common, when suction drainage tubes, particularly in axillary surgery, is removed prematurely,

- lymphoedema — which is rare in an early postoperative period but, may develop later due to low-grade infection and obstruction to lymph flow. Proper and prompt antibiotic therapy must be given, if there is any sign of infection, with advice to avoid trauma to hand or arm. It may occur as a result of surgery or radiotherapy causing much of the distress, pain and discomfort. Limb exercise, massage and compression bandaging may be helpful to relieve the symptoms.

- nerve damage — involvement of intercostal and axillary nerves may result in pain and can develop weakness in the shoulder muscles and even paralysis of the arm.

By Radiotherapy :

Radiotherapy is a localised form of treatment used to treat areas where surgical procedures (for example — supraclavicular lymph nodes and internal mammary nodes, etc.) are difficult to perform. It also plays an important role in the palliation of recurrent disease following wide local excision or quadrantectomy or mastectomy, in locally advanced cancer and in areas of a high incidence of an occult lymph node metastasis when the disease has already reached the axilla. It should not be given to the surgically cleared axilla because it increases the possibility of distressing postoperative lymphoedema.

Usually, the breast cancer presents itself as a painless lump and originates where there is maximum volume of breast tissue. The highest incidences are observed in the upper and outer quadrant — 45 percent, central area — 30 percent, lower and an outer quadrant — 15 percent and lowest in a lower-inner quadrant — 10 percent). Radiotherapy is normally given in fractional doses over a period of three to five weeks depending on the stages of the disease and size of the tumour. The effectiveness of the combined surgery and radiotherapy improves survival rates by eradicating loco-regional disease before it has the chance to spread in various places. A careful selection of women, with appropriate location and size of the tumour, usually smaller than four centimetres, with the size of the breast, can also achieve a remarkable success rate by radiotherapy.

The incidence of side effects following radiotherapy has been greatly reduced with technological improvement in the modern machine and in the method of delivery of radiation. The side effects can be further reduced, if the woman is fully informed and warned before the treatment (for example — fear, depression, nausea, lethargy and tiredness, etc.). Local skin reactions as redness, tight feeling of the skin and there may be a stiffness in the shoulder joint etc. are more often seen either during or soon after the treatment. Risk of developing cardiac damage, pneumonitis, oesophagitis, nerve damage to brachial plexus and radiation necrosis to rib or clavicle or humerus is less common than they used to be. Palliative radiotherapy has got very little or no value for a visceral metastasis but helps in relieving pain from a skeletal metastasis.

By Chemotherapy :

The aim of chemotherapy in the management of the breast cancer should be the highest clinical and pathological response rate for a longer duration with least short-term and long-term toxicity. It can be given either to women with established metastatic disease or as a prophylaxis to women at high risk of developing recurrent cancer after a mastectomy (for example — those with an axillary node metastasis). It is more effective than endocrine (hormone) therapy in younger women who have rapidly progressing tumours, an extensive visceral metastasis (for examples — liver, lungs and the brain etc.), oestrogen-receptor negative tumours and even after the failure of previous hormone therapy. In general, both the response rate and the duration of response are lower with a single agent than with combined agents. Therefore combined, regimes should always be used after a mastectomy to inhibit growth of micro-metastasis. Since all the agents are used, is somewhat immunosuppressive because for being cytotoxic, their use is not without risk. In Britain, most commonly used chemotherapeutic agents are cyclophosphamide, methotrexate and flurouracil in various combinations, preferably with a corticosteroid to suppress endogenous adrenal function. Other chemotherapeutic agents, such as, chlorumbucil, vincristin, dexorubicin and melphalan have limited use and should be used only those experienced in cancer chemotherapy. Some units prefer to use dexorubicin in premenopausal women with a high risk of developing recurrent breast cancer. The systemic form of therapy in women with breast cancer is a complex process. The disease also differs from woman to woman and with the various agents, mostly in various combinations, may be appropriate under certain circumstances.

The most commonly noticed side effects are nausea, vomiting, lethargy, bone marrow depression, diarrhoea, infertility, risk of infection, early menopause and hair loss.

Today, continuous research and development of new treatment, experience and judgement in clinical practice and constant improvement in the relative services make it possible for many breast cancer women to live longer and may even cure some women.

By Hormone Therapy :

The aim of hormone therapy is either to reduce symptoms or to delay the process of advancement of the cancer cells and thus prolonging the life expectancy. It can be given in combination with radiotherapy when the disease recurs following a mastectomy and when the disease is advanced so that the surgery cannot be performed — only givens as a palliative treatment. Recently, hormone therapy has been extended to women with large (operable) tumours with an attempt to reduce the size of the tumour first, thus making it convenient for surgery and suitable for breast conservation.

Breast cancer can be treated by a wide range of hormone treatments either by removal of both ovaries (called bilateral oophorectomy) rather than by irradiation of the ovaries in premenopausal women or an antioestrogenic drug — tamoxifen in both pre and post menopausal women. Most of the breast cancers are heterogeneous — with mixture of oestrogen receptor positive and oestrogen receptor negative cells. The response to any hormone therapy depends on the presence of oestrogen receptor cells in the tumour. Therefore, any absences of oestrogen receptor cells inhibit cell division and hence the tumour growth. Women with oestrogen receptor positive tumours respond to hormone therapy in about 60 percent of cases whereas less than 10 percent in oestrogen receptor negative tumours.

Removals of the ovaries benefit the treatment of recurrent or advanced breast cancer in women under 50 and the remission can lasts up to two years or more but not without any side effects — menopausal symptoms.

Androgens, either as testosterone propionate or one of the anabolic steroid, such as, durabolin, usually given by injection method, can also provide similar results like the oophorectomy. It is the treatment of choice for premenopausal women although it can be given to women of all ages. The most common side effect is virilism, which may be distressing in some women.

Oestrogens in a high dosage were standard treatment in women in advanced age — 70 or more for breast cancer before tamoxifen. It should never be given to premenopausal women with breast cancer as they may stimulate tumour growth. Nausea, vomiting, vaginal bleeding and fluid retention is the common side effects. Since the introduction of tamoxifen both oestrogens and androgens are not used for the treatment of breast cancer.

At present, tamoxifen is the treatment of choice for breast cancer all over the world. It is most effective and widely used as hormone therapy in women with breast cancer of all age groups. The standard dose is ten milligrams twice a day by mouth. It is more effective in long term therapy, but five years' treatment better than two years treatment, than a short term, moreover reduces the risk of developing contralateral breast cancer by about 40 percent. A remarkable benefit can be achieved in women with tumours rich in oestrogen receptor cells than in tumours with poor oestrogen receptor cells. Although it is well-tolerated, the most common side effects, such as, hot flushes, loss of a libido, nausea, vomiting, vaginal dryness, menstrual disturbances, weights gains are often seen, especially in premenopausal women. These side effects can be counteracted by appropriate therapy — vaginal dryness by nonhormonal product, either K-Y jelly or replen, hot flushes by clonidine and menopausal symptoms by evening primrose oil, etc.

Most recent studies show treatment with raloxifen (a selective oestrogen positive receptor) is found to be very effective and promising in the prevention of breast cancer. A treatment with raloxifen, more than three years substantially reduces the risk of invasive breast cancer with no increase in the incidence of endometrial cancer. An increased risk of a deep vein thrombosis or pulmonary embolism also noticed with raloxifen. Hormone therapy in combination with chemotherapy can cause fatigue, lethargy, infection (oral mucositis), neutropenia and the most distressing side effect — alopecia.

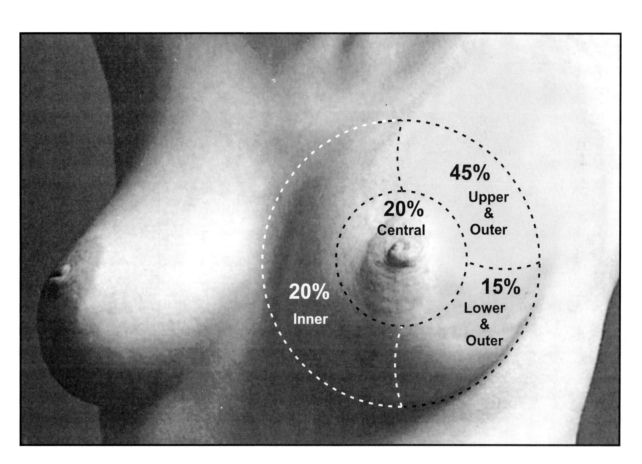

Usual location and incidence of breast cancer.

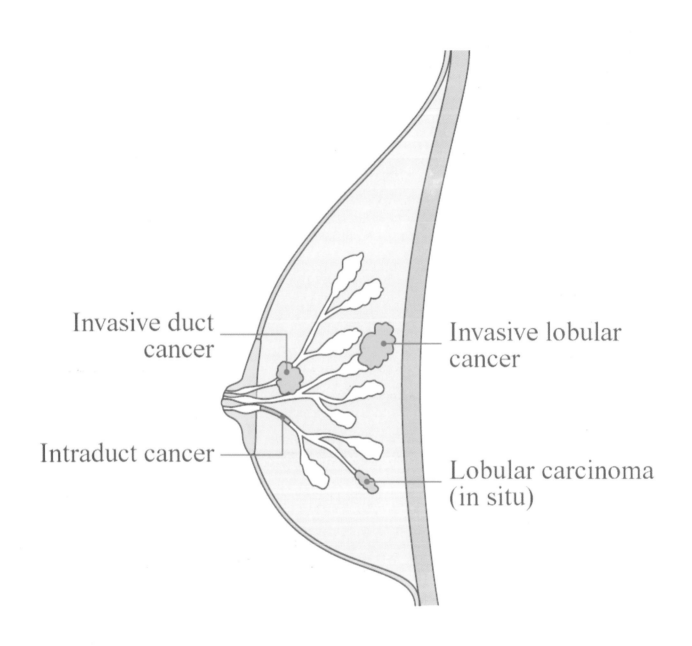

Invasive duct cancer

Invasive lobular cancer

Intraduct cancer

Lobular carcinoma (in situ)

Classification of breast cancer :
Non-Invasive (in situ) form - Cancer cells remain within the basement membrane.
Invasive form - Cancer cells spread outside the basement membrane and surrounding tissue.

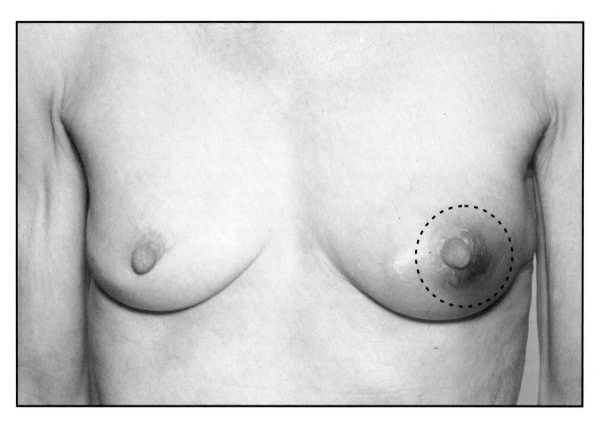

Carcinoma of the left breast.

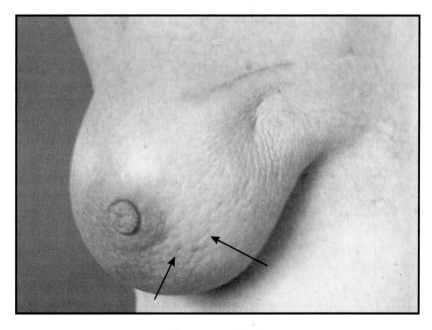

Peau d'orange of the breast.
Note - changes on breast skin surface - skin dimpling due to cancer above

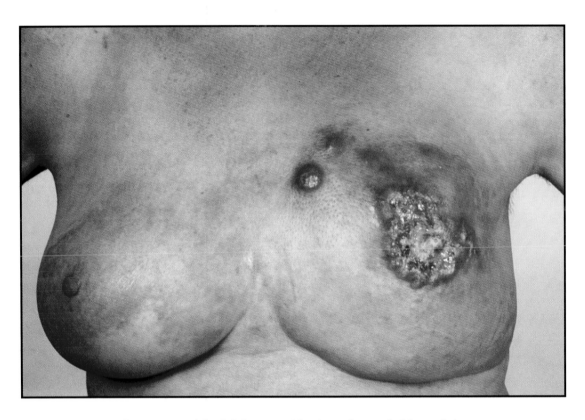

Carcinoma of the left breast with ulceration and skin nodule.

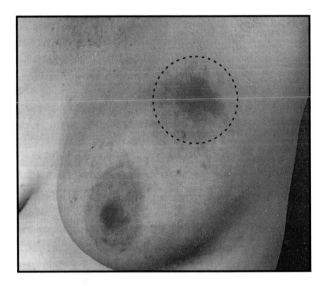

Inflammatory carcinoma of the left breast -
Diagnosis confirmed by neddle aspiration and culture.
Note : bruised area.

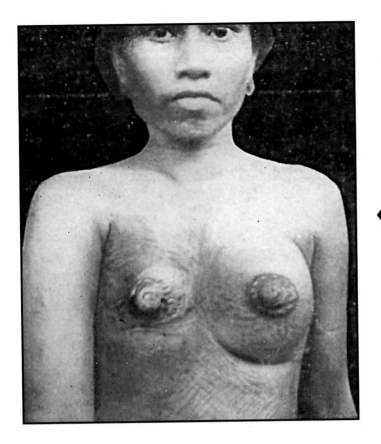

Bilateral carcinoma
of the breast.
The right one
was first affected.

*(Permission given to reproduce
this photograph - by Dr. S. Das)*

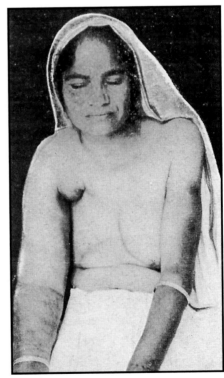

Oedematous right arm
(lymphoedema)
developed after
radical mastectomy.

*(Permission given to reproduce
this photograph - by Dr. S. Das)*

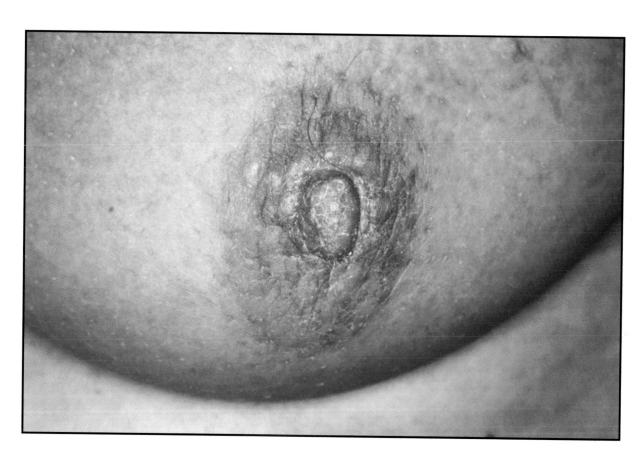

Radiation dermatitis.
(Nipple and surrounding area)

CHAPTER 13

Breast Cancer and Oral Contraceptives

The breast cancer is a major health problem throughout the world, especially in developed countries. Combined oral contraceptives have been available in America for clinical use since 1959. During the last 40 years, combined oral contraceptives have been widely used in many countries of the world including in Britain to avoid unwanted pregnancies or for pacing pregnancies. The exact cause of breast cancer is unknown but a harmful biological effect is observed after a long period of exposure with most carcinogenous products. Any growth and differentiation of the breast tissues are regulated by many of factors including steroid hormones, such as, oestrogen and progesterone. Therefore, administration of combined oral contraceptives could have an effect on breast carcinogenesis. Oestrogen causes proliferation of the breast tissue and would be expected to increase the risk of breast cancer by stimulating growth of stem and intermediate cells. Progesterone, on the other hand, causes not only alveolar cell growth in the oestrogen-primed breast but also differentiation. Thus, the use of combined oral contraceptives and their effect on the development of breast cancer, however small, whether it is harmful or beneficial, may be the basis on the pathogenesis of this devastating disease. Over the past 40 years combined oral contraceptives have become one of the most intensively studied drugs all over the world and the results reported to date are inconclusive. The basic question whether there is any definite relationship between combined oral contraceptives and the development of the breast cancer, is remain to be the same.

During the last 30 years, two very important changes, such as, chemical formulation of the pills leading towards smaller and smaller doses of active hormones and the increasing use by younger women have been noticed. Thus, the modern combined oral contraceptives are as effective as the earlier high oestrogen pills with very little carcinogenic effect. To date, most published studies covering various data, have come to the conclusion that certain factors have close relationships than other in the development of breast cancer. The various data, such as, different patterns of chemical formulation, family history of breast cancer, menopausal status, histories of benign breast disease, personal habit and racial factor, etc. are included in these studies. So far there has been a disturbing lack of consistency in the results between women with strong family history (for example - mother, sister and daughter) and susceptible group of women.

In summary —

- All women irrespective of their ages and the couples, if any, should have thoroughly explained the merits and side effects of the oral contraceptives. They should be given sufficient time at the clinic as well as home for decision making.

- A full medical and family history and clinical examination must be carried out by medical professionals at the outset followed by review facility.

- All women, especially young women, should undertake regular breast self-examination whether on or off the pill.

- Any persistent lump or nodularity in the breast must be reported to the medical professionals for confirmation and intervention, earlier rather than later.

The woman or the couple, thus reducing the mortality and morbidity of breast cancer from combined oral contraceptive use, must make final decisions.

CHAPTER 14

Breast Cancer and Pregnancy

The incidence of breast cancer during pregnancy is about 1 to 2 percent of all breast cancers with the average age of the women being 30 to 35 years. Lately, a shift in the incidence of pregnancy in the reproductive age group of women has been identified because more and more women are delaying childbearing into their late 30's or early 40's where usually breast cancer can be more common.

The diagnosis of breast cancer during pregnancy is often confused, delayed and even difficult to identify especially small obscure tumours in the breasts even by experienced medical personnel because of normal enlargement of breast and lumpiness. This means, that woman is not easily subject to any immediate diagnostic procedures, thus allowing the tumour to grow further locally or distant by spreading to axillary nodes until they are well-advanced.

Some mammograms, although the foetal radiation exposure is small, are not a reliable method of diagnosis of breast cancer during pregnancy because it substantially reduces the quality of the picture due to increased blood supply and water content. Histological diagnosis, by way of excision biopsy, which should be carried out with great care to avoid infection and disruption of milk ducts, remains the diagnostic tests of choice during pregnancy.

If the diagnosis is confirmed during the first and second trimesters of pregnancy, surgery is the treatment of choice. The radiotherapy and chemotherapy increase the risk of congenital foetal malformations, chromosomal damage, growth disturbances, mental retardation and childhood malignancy, especially, leukaemia.

During the third trimester, the breast cancer can be treated either by immediate surgery, provided the pregnancy has reached the stage of foetal viability or by delaying for a short period to allow the pregnancy to continue until the viable stage is reached while monitoring the tumour very closely. With the improvements in the standard management technique, neonatal complications, such as, cerebral haemorrhage, respiratory distress syndrome, feeding difficulties, anaemia and jaundice etc., can be substantially reduced once the pregnancy reaches 30 to 32 weeks of gestation. Surgery should be performed without any further delay if the tumour shows any sign of an increase in size during the monitoring period. Obviously, the decisions which should be a team decision — by surgeon, obstetrician, oncologist, neonatal paediatrician and above all the woman concerned, as to the timing is crucial.

Following breast cancer, any woman considering a pregnancy should have extensive counselling because of the high incidence of a relapse rate — 80 percent, during the first two years. Women with evidence of axillary node involvement or evidence of recurrent disease, should be strongly discouraged for further pregnancy as the chance of her long term survival as well as the pregnancy reaching a viable stage will be greatly shortened.

CHAPTER 15

Breast Cancer and Hormone Replacement Therapy

The menopause, which occurs in all women, is a physiological event and often associated with various distressing symptoms due to lack of the sexual hormone (oestrogen). The age at which the menopause occurs varies greatly, the average being 45 to 48 years, so the symptoms can be — mild, moderate and severe in intensity, a few per month to several per hour in frequency. At present, average female life expectancy is about 80 years. Thus, women can expect to live about 30 years of her life in postmenopausal oestrogen deficient state. The vast majority of postmenopausal groups aged over 50 years usually suffer from - hot flushes, depression, dry skin, irritability, night sweating, insomnia, mood swing, episodes of tearfulness, poor memory, lack of concentration, etc. Women with advancing age and the loss of socially desirable characteristics, such as, youth and beauty, energy, healthy looking skin, and feelings of well-being, now have the choice of having a hormone replacement therapy (HRT) to alleviate their symptoms.

Before starting any hormone replacement therapy, whether natural or synthetic preparation, a full medical history, examination, and discussion about the therapy, especially benefits and side effects, should be explained by the medical personnel, so that the woman should be in full possession of facts and understand the risks. A regular annual review and good communication between the woman and her doctor and, if necessary, with the breast specialist may reduce the risk of developing breast cancer with hormone replacement therapy.

Breast cancer, which is common after the menopause, is a hormonal cancer. It is the biggest killer of women aged 40 to 50, especially when the woman has a first degree relative, such as, mother, sister, and daughter with breast cancer as well as a history of a surgically proven benign breast disease. At the menopause, breast involution follows due to loss of ovarian function. Thus, there is reduction in the amount of glandular tissue and relative predominance of connective tissue. With hormone replacement therapy, breast density increases, making it more difficult to detect breast cancer.

Hormone replacement therapy can be administered in various formulations, such as, tablets, patches, implants, gels, vaginal pessaries and cream. Women, who have had a hysterectomy, only need to have oestrogen, while women with wombs must have combined (oestrogen and progesterone) therapy. The side effects can be greatly reduced by careful selection of women. Hormone replacement therapy also helps to protect from endometrial and ovarian cancer, heart disease, Alzheimer's disease, and osteoporosis but the possibility of a thromboembolic phenomenon (a deep vein thrombosis and pulmonary embolism) must not be ignored.

During the last decade, several better-designed case controlled study been published and the results are contradictory. Some reported breast cancer might be a serious problem with oestrogen alone or with combined preparations but others did not. However, it is important to establish whether there is an increased risk with higher doses and over a longer period with hormone therapy or not. Most recent study with hormone replacement therapy suggests that the risk of breast cancer is be increased by up to 50 percent after ten to 15 years of use. Therefore, with present knowledge breast cancer risk continues to increase with advancing age and uninterrupted prolonged use of hormone therapy, say more than ten years. Although, most postmenopausal women are at risk from heart disease, and osteoporosis than breast cancer itself, perhaps, time and future research on any form of new treatment, particularly on meditation, homeopathy, acupuncture, hydrotherapy and diet etc. may alter the view of present form of hormone therapy.

CHAPTER 16

Breast Reconstruction Surgery

The aim of breast reconstruction surgery, especially following breast cancer, is to create a normal, natural (soft in consistency with slight mobility) and comfortable breasts as near as possible to their earlier shape whether dressed or undressed. Reconstructive breast surgery, which is popular in America, is becoming more fashionable and acceptable in Britain. There are various reasons for reconstructive procedures either medical or surgical or both. Women, who request breast augmentation or reduction or uplifting, have a significantly different problem from those, who had lost their breast because of cancer. Following breast cancer surgery (for example — a mastectomy, extensive local excision, etc.), the demand for breast reconstruction's either on the affected breast with an implant or on the natural breast (augmentation or reduction) to preserve symmetrical identity has been increasing for the past decade.

Breast reconstruction happens in selected women where prophylactic removal of the opposite breast is recommended as well as following an accidental injury. The reconstructive procedures, which depend on individual preferences, can be done immediately after the cancer surgery or delayed for several weeks to months following mastectomies. It is very difficult to achieve perfect symmetry in size, shape, and nipple-areolar position of the breast and some mobility and natural consistency. These characteristics not only depend on the amount and type of the remaining skin but also the size, shape, and texture of the opposite breast.

Immediate reconstruction procedure is ideal for a healthy, well-informed woman with small breasts and localised disease. It is safe, there is less risk of local and systemic recurrence and it is not a contra-indication of adjuvant chemotherapy or radiation. It also saves time and cost of second time surgery. Most women prefer this procedure which gives them better cosmetic results and also reduces psychological trauma.

The immediate reconstruction procedure can be performed by placement of a prosthesis (a silicon gel implant) or insertion of a tissue expander or insertion of a flap of skin and muscle with or without prosthesis (implant) where necessary.

The insertion of a tissue expander, which is a temporary device, is to stretch the skin of the anterior chest wall and muscle over a period of weeks, if not months. It is placed under pectoralis major and part of serratus anterior, and rectus abdominis muscle and inflated with saline through a subcutaneous valve. This method can be used both in immediate and delayed procedures of reconstruction surgery works best in women with small breasts and those who have not received any radiation therapy previously. It is a less complicated procedure and is often associated with discomfort of the chest wall and ribs rather than myocutaneous flap method. When the skin is stretched at a desired level the expander is removed and a permanent silicon gel implant is placed.

The delayed reconstruction procedure allows the breast time to settle especially, following radiotherapy which may interfere with sound healing and skin graft, if any, and may help to reconstruct the nipple areolar complex with good results. In the myocutaneous flap method, two most common myocutaneous flaps, either latissimai dorsi muscles with overlying skin from the upper back together with its blood supply or lower abdominal flap and skins based on the transverse rectus abdominis muscle with its blood supply, are used. Women, who have had the radiotherapies are often better served with myocutaneous flaps with or without prosthesis, which provide skin and muscle replacement.

In the latissimai dorsi flap technique, usually the silicon gel implant is fixed underneath the skin and muscle and an excellent cosmetic result can be achieved, especially for those looking for larger breasts. There may be a problem in healing and some weakness in the arm or shoulder when the transplanted muscle is combined with a tissue expander. At the same time an additional scar at the back cannot be avoided. In transverse rectus abdominis flap technique, an implant may not be necessary because of the added advantage of an unwanted abdominal bulge. It also helps to keep the figure in shape. Although, there are no further problems with capsular contraction, a greater risk of graft failure does exist. Other complications, such as, skin and fat necrosis, weakness in the abdominal wall may lead to a hernia.

The final problem is producing a nipple-areolar complex. The reconstruction procedure should be deferred to allow the breast time to settle. The areola can be simulated by taking a full thickness dark disk of skin from the upper inner thigh after careful removal of hair follicles from the inner aspect of the graft or in some situations part of the contralateral areola can be used. Tattooing techniques have also been tried for areolar reconstruction but it may have to be repeated if the colour fades away. The nipple reconstruction can be made by using local tissue to produce nipple prominence or by sharing contralateral nipple or by nipple prosthesis to provide additional nipple projection and shape and colour.

Augmentation :

The aim of breast augmentation is to enhance self-image by increasing the bulk of the breasts featuring uplifting, fullness, roundness, good nipple position and projection, and symmetrical in proportion to the other body dimensions and to the general quality of the build. Abnormally small size breasts and postpartum volume loss of the breasts are the typical group of women seeking advice for breast augmentation procedure. A limited number of women may require such procedure for cosmetic and social reasons because of wide local excisions have been performed on the breast for breast cancer. Women with abnormally small size breasts, which may be partial or total, unilateral or bilateral, are usually deficient both in skin and underlying breast tissue, often similar to those in women with a mastectomy. Normally, most women's breasts are asymmetric, the left usually being larger than the right breast. Thus, sometimes, it is difficult to achieve perfect symmetries even under best circumstances including nipple height, diameter, projection and sensation. Whatever the situation, women must understand this perplexity and be sure that it is she, who wants the augmentation procedure — not someone else. The basic impulse must come from the women.

Before contemplating such breast augmentation procedures, women should consult a plastic surgeon, either privately or under the National Health Service, who is experienced and widely known in the field. Disfigurement by clumsy, inexperienced surgeons not only costs time, energy and money, but also causes psychological trauma and bitterness. A proper medical history, especially family history with first degree breast cancer — mother, sister, and daughter, history of any other breast problems, clinical examination, full information on technique, various types of implant materials available for such procedure, and their advantage and disadvantages, postoperative complications and follow-up services are essential.

In the past, various types of implant materials, such as, ivalon sponges made of polyvinyl, gel-filled silicon bags with a teardrop shaped fixation patches on the posterior wall, and saline inflatable implants were used for breast augmentation surgery. The increasing number of unsatisfactory results and postoperative complications, such as, hardness, asymmetry, irregularity in the breast, wide spread incidences of infection, leakage of the gel, sinus formation, haematoma and painful capsular contracture, makes them unsuitable for such procedure.

At present, the most popularly used implant is polyurethane-covered a silicon gel prosthesis. Although debatable, it neither increases nor decreases a woman's risk of developing breast cancer in the future. It is preferred by most surgeons, acceptable by most women and has a minimum side effect with good results. A full preoperative discussion for suitability of individual incisions, such as, axillary incision — cosmetically appealing, circum-areolar incision — well disguised popular one, and inframammary crease incision — most popular and safest one, should play an important role in the success of the procedure as well as satisfaction to the woman.

Reduction :

Breast reduction is aimed to reduce disproportionately large, heavy weight, and pendulous breasts while improving shape and configuration including size of the areola and nipple thus lifting confidence, body image, overall appearance, comfort and health. Women with hypertrophied breasts, often encounter various problems, such as —

- **weight bearing pain** — usually in the neck, shoulders and back, and grooving of the shoulder skin from the pressure of the bra-straps due to heavy weight, restriction of physical activity — particularly in running and taking part in various sports,
- **pulmonary difficulties** — aggravation of asthma or a chronic obstructive airways disease symptoms,
- **skin rashes** — often associated with infection and odour due to continuous friction and poor air circulation of the breasts underneath,
- **artificial posture** — usually they adopt a stooping posture to mask apparent size of their breasts,
- **colourful clothing** — by wearing dark coloured clothes and a large size.

Above all, the most important effect is psychological distress, especially in young women. Abnormal breast enlargements, either unilateral or bilateral, often seen at puberty, are the commonest causes of distress and embarrassment in most women relating to body images. In some women such enlargement may also occur at the time of pregnancy as well as at the menopause. Some women who have undergone a mastectomy have chosen to wear a smaller and lighter prosthesis, may also seek a reduction procedure on their unduly large remaining breast.

Reduction mammoplasty considerably improves quality of life, boosts morale and should be more easily available, although it is not always possible, to reconstruct a breast like a mirror image of the natural breast. The degree of reduction depends on general stature and desirability of a good cosmetic result. In reduction mammoplasty not only the size and shape of the breasts but also the positioning of the nipple and its functional capability (future breast-feeding in some cases) especially in younger women together with the size of the areola can pose problems. To achieve a rewarding and pleasing result, like any other surgical procedures and before consenting to such treatment, women should have full explanation and understand the whole affair, such as, various types of operations in practice today, benefits and side effects. Above all, careful selection made by the woman and the individual surgeon's experience and preferences are equally important to avoid disfigurement and bitterness for the rest of her life.

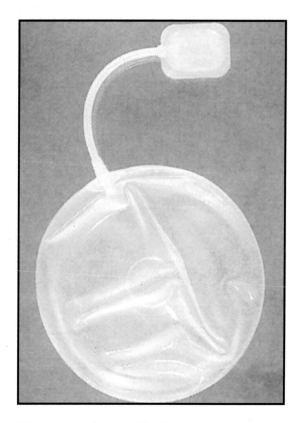

Tissue expander used for breast reconstruction.

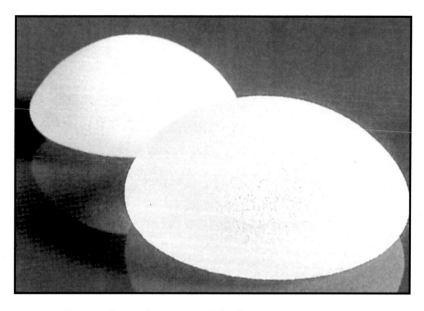

Textured prostheses - used for breast reconstruction.

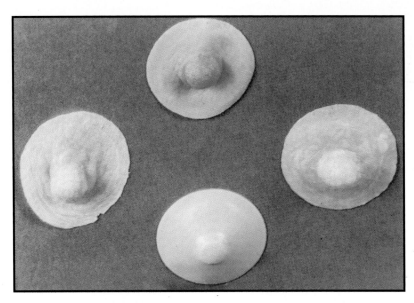

Customised prosthetic nipple (top)
and other three commercially available ones.

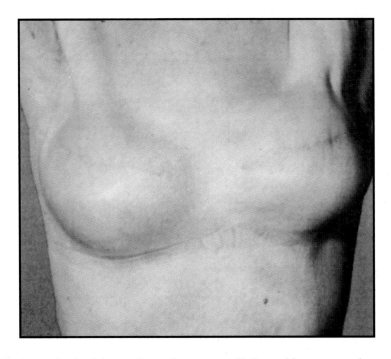

Patient who had immediate placement of bilateral breast prostheses.

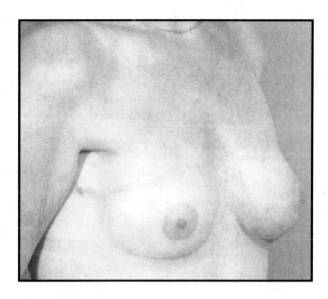

Breast reconstruction with permanent prosthesis
after previous tissue expansion.
(Nipple complex has also been reconstructed).

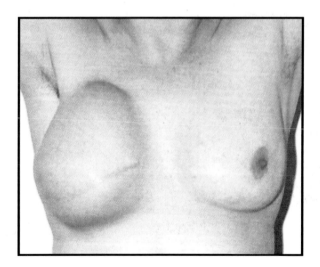

Patient with tissue expander in situ
that is overexpanded.

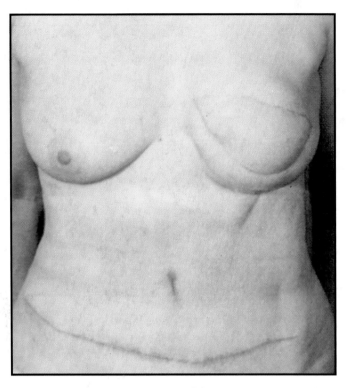

Patient who underwent breast reconstruction with
transverse rectus abdominis muscle (TRAM) flap;
Note - large abdominal scar.

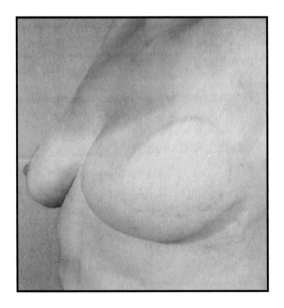
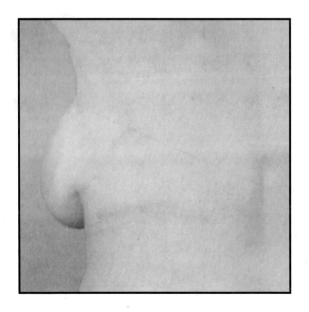

Patient who underwent immediate latissimus dorsi myocutaneous flap reconstruction :
(left) side view showing ptosis that can be achieved; (right) scar on back.

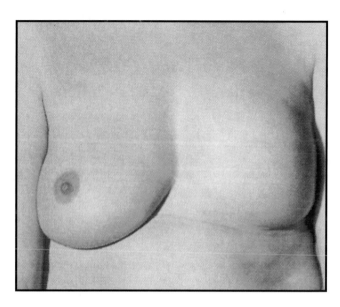

Breast reconstruction with tissue expansion and prosthesis;
Note - lack of potsis in reconstructed breast (left).

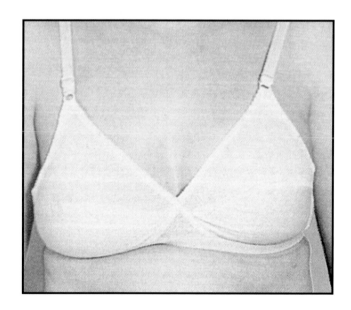

Note - lack of potsis is hidden when a bra is worn
by above patient.

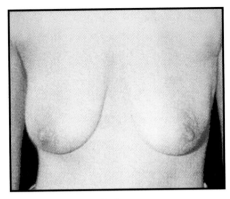

Before

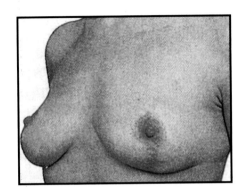

After

Reconstruction of the breasts (lifting).

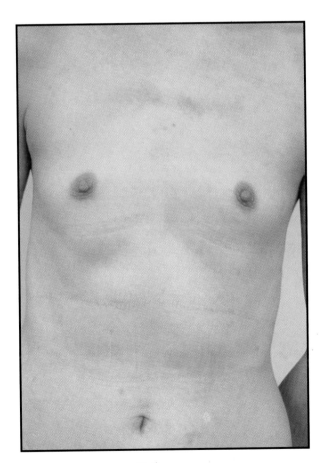

Before

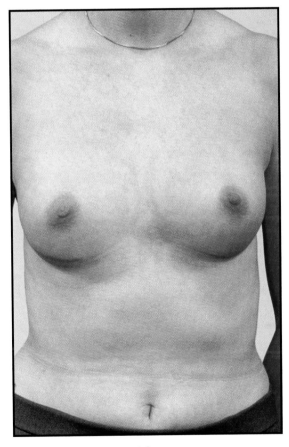

After

Reconstruction of the breasts (augmentation)..

Reconstruction of the breasts (reduction).

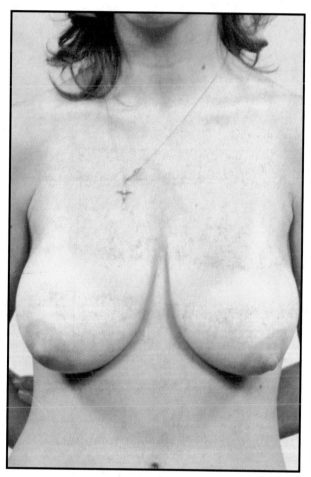

Before

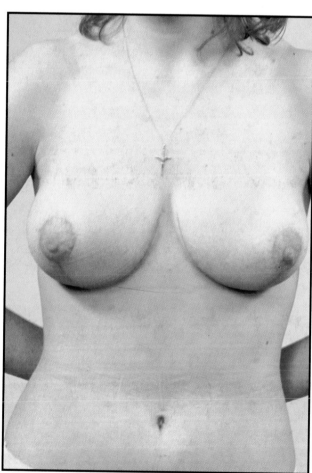

After

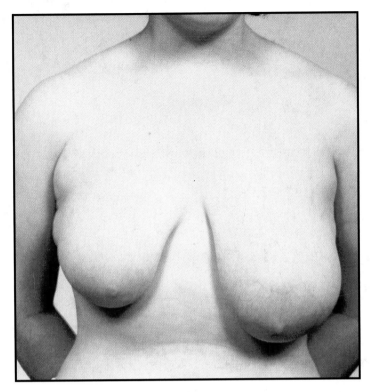

Before

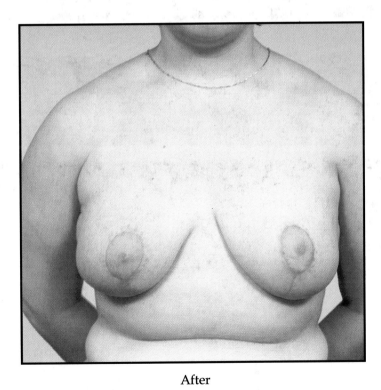

After

Asymmetry of the breasts.

CHAPTER 17

Breast Cancer and Metastasis

The breast is richly supplied with blood vessels and lymph capillaries and is linked with neighbouring structures and thus plays an important part in the spread of malignant disease. Normally, regional lymph nodes are involved — axillary nodes being first and commonest, followed by internal mammary nodes, and then supraclavicular nodes. A distant metastatic lesion normally occurs through the vascular system.

Axillary Lymph Nodes :

The incidences of metastatic breast cancer in the axillary lymph nodes are as high as 50 percent in women with operable breast cancer. The axillary nodal involvement is directly related to the size of the primary tumour and its location - higher in the central and outer half than in the inner and middle half of the breast. The metastasis, first seen at the lower nodes of the anterior axillary chain then spread to the middle and upper nodes. Thus, the axillary nodal status, important single factor to indicate survival incidence for breast cancer and also dictates future treatment plans.

Women, who are with four or more histologically positive axillary nodes', increase the incidence of an internal mammary node involvement and distant metastasis. Therefore, women with positive axillary nodes following dissection procedure should have a radical radiotherapy, whereas women with negative nodes require no further treatment other than watch policy. By adopting this method of treatment recurrence rates can be reduced.

Internal Mammary Nodes :

The location of the primary tumour — inner and central areas, and histologically proved a positive axillary lymph node enhances the chance of a metastasis to the internal mammary lymph nodes. Most women with positive internal mammary nodes have significantly poorer survival rates due to involvement of wider areas as well as from the side effects of her treatment.

Supraclavicular Nodes :

A supraclavicular metastasis usually occurs following extensive involvement of either axillary nodes or internal mammary nodes or both. It can occur in an isolation manner when the cancer cells affect skins of the upper half of the breast.

Distant Metastasis :

Women with a positive axillary nodes and supraclavicular metastasis are most commonly involved with a distant metastasis, first through the lymphatic system to the regional lymph nodes and then through the blood circulation to distant sites — clavicle, humerus, ribs, lungs, liver and brain etc.

A distant metastasis may present as bone pain, pathological fractures, general malaise and weakness, lethargy, nausea, vomiting, constipation, pleural effusion, breathlessness, anorexia, weight loss, jaundice, an increase in intracranial pressure, headache, and various neurological symptoms (for examples, fits, speech and movement disturbances) depending on the affected sites. Most women with locally recurrent breast cancer, although the incidence is low, following surgery and radiotherapy can be salvaged by further surgery — not by radiotherapy, if this treatment has been given earlier. Systemic therapy should be advocated when the recurrence occurs at different distant sites. Therefore, an adequate and effective treatment at the beginning is the best strategy; to prevent the recurrence of advanced breast cancer in either local or distant metastasis.

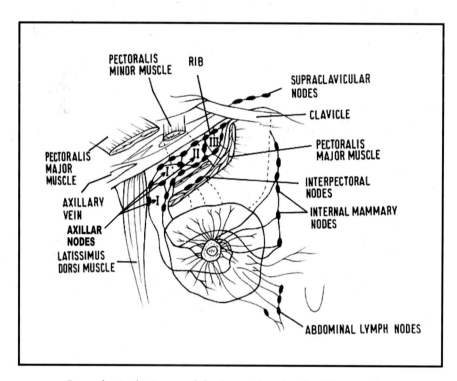

Lymphatic drainage of the breast levels of axillary nodes.

CHAPTER 18

Breast Cancer Follow-up

The aim of follow-up clinic following breast cancer surgery is to improve the quality and standard of the woman's life, to avoid recurrence, and to re-establish confidence. Follow-up is a standard practice in most centres following any form of surgical intervention or after any form of special therapy (for example, radiotherapy, chemotherapy etc.), but the duration depends on the primary condition. The cancer follow-up period can be extended between ten and 15 years depending on the stage of the disease at diagnosis. Routine follow-ups are normally carried out at the hospital outpatients' clinic, mainly a special breast clinic, but in some centres where strong primary care is available, a shared responsibility between the general practitioner and the specialist at the hospital can be arranged. The recommended follow-up schedule varies from centre to centre after the diagnosis and individual need. Normally, it is every three months for the first year, every six months for the year two to five and every year thereafter. Apart from history taking, physical examinations, blood tests, and some mammograms — every 12 to 36 months, is usually done in some centres depending on initial treatment and age of the woman. Other investigations, if required, will also be carried out accordingly.

CHAPTER 19

Breast Cancer and Psychological Effect

Most women find either the threat to the breast or loss of a breast extremely distressing and this has a devastating effect not only on herself but also those closest to her. Usually, breast cancer afflicts when the women are most needed by their family, especially if they have some young children or a husband with stressful and demanding jobs, or perhaps the woman just started a top job of her career or just planning for a long and happy retirement life. Most women also find it is most stressful and difficult time of her life waiting for the results of her tests. During this period, there are lots of thoughts are going through her mind, such as, loss of femininity, the damaging effect on her relationship, fears of recurrence of the disease, unable to cope with the domestic and other duties. The side effects of various treatments, body image, progressive pain and disability leading to death, etc., making her more susceptible to develop anxiety state and depressive illness. Most women with such illness usually show signs of irritability, insomnia, inability to enjoy herself, impaired concentration and mood change etc.

Growing awareness of these psycho-social problems led to the development of the various supportive therapies for the women and their families. Supportive therapy may be offered formally or informally by various health professionals or by lay volunteers including a breast cancer sufferer themselves or by a wide variety of either local or national self-help groups.

Depending on the severity of the problems, women can be treated either by her general practitioner or by the specialist unit at the hospital. Nearly, 30 percent of women with breast cancers develop anxiety state and depressive illness during the first year of diagnosis and 20 to 30 percent of women develop body image and sexual relationship difficulties after a mastectomy operation. A cheerful, optimistic approach, better understanding about each other's views and truthful explanations about the diagnosis and treatment and emotional support play an important role in the satisfactory outcome, if not, full recovery. Mild anxiety state can be treated by either with anxiolytics — a benzodiazepine or with an anti-psychotic drug — a phenothiazine group. This type of treatment should be given for a short period to avoid any drug dependency. Propranolol, a betablocker, can be helpful where somatic symptoms of anxiety, such as, mood changes, insomnia, irritability, etc., is predominant. Antidepressants (for examples — dothiepin) are the drugs of choice and can be given for a longer period for depressive illness without causing any dependency problems. Persistence and severe forms of anxiety state and depressive illness should be treated with specialist care at the hospital.

Psycho-educational, which is an extension of postoperative physiotherapy teaching practice, must be continued at home after discharge from the hospital. It helps with relaxation technique, in improving coping skills, to enhance self-image problems including sexual difficulties and also helps in reducing pain symptoms. The ideas of these exercises are also to improve arm and shoulder mobility and reduce the risk of development of lymphoedema. These exercises (for examples — hair-brushing, bra-fastening, wall-reaching, arm-swinging, squeezing and relaxing hand, rope-pulley exercise, rope-string exercise, bean-bag exercise, back-drying exercise, etc.) helps them to return as soon as possible to their previous daily active life. Psycho-social interventions not only improve quality of women's life but also extend the survival rate.

CHAPTER 20

Breast Cancer in Male

Breast cancer is the commonest form of cancer in female but men are not immune to this.

Simple self-observation by men can help to detect cancer at its early, more treatable stages, leading to improved chances of survival. Men are less likely to report any changes of their breasts because of simple ignorance or pride or embarrassment. Normally, during the adolescence period, young men can have an excess of the oestrogen hormone rather than the usual testosterone, which can stimulates their breast tissue to form a well-developed breast as in women. This development is called gynaecomastia, usually a benign condition, which requires only careful observation and medical advice at some point. Young men with well-developed breasts not only feel embarrassed but also run the risk of being a potential target for abuse. Surgical removal is the choice of treatment in such cases. For any reason, if it is due to some form of hormone therapy, a with drawl of such therapy will be sufficient for it to go back to its original condition.

From adolescence onwards men should regularly check their nipples for signs of

- any swelling underneath, especially painless swelling,
- any redness, soreness, cracking, or any blistering,
- any inversion,
- any discharge, especially blood,
- any lasting irritation or pain.

The main causes of breast cancers are the same as in women.

Age :

Chances are higher as men grow older.

Family History :

Histories of first degree breast cancer in the family, such as, mother, sister and brother enhances the incidence of male breast cancer.

Chromosomal Abnormality :

Men with an extra sex chromosome not producing some sufficient amounts of testosterone are susceptible to have a breast cancer than others.

Other Factors :

Diet, Obesity, lack of exercise, etc. may be the other contributory factors in the development of breast cancer.

As far as the treatment is concerned, there is no difference in the management of breast cancer in men as in women. It is either in single form or a combination form consists of surgery, radiotherapy, chemotherapy and hormone therapy depending on the stages at diagnosis.

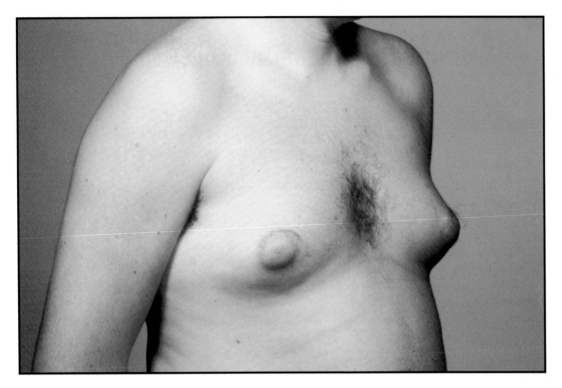

Gynaecomastia

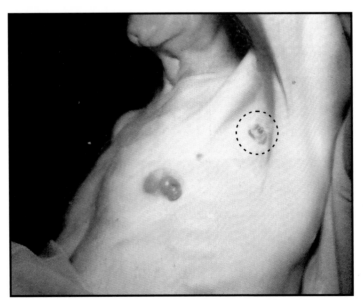

Carcinoma of the male breast. Infiltration of the skin can be seen.
The black mark on skin of the axilla is directly over a palpable and
obviously involved axillary node.

INDEX

Breast Cancer Information and Help line

CANADA :

Canadian Cancer Society.
URL: http://www.cancer.ca/
Tel... 1 888 939 - 3333   (toll-free)
Email: info@cis.cancer.ca

EUROPE :

TeleSCAN: Telematic Services in Cancer.
URL: http://www.telescan.nki.nl/

GREECE :

Hellenic Cancer Society.
URL: http://www.addgr.com/org/hc/

INDIA :

Mastectomy Association of India (M.I.A.).
Santosh Handa, A-38, Meera Bagh, Outer ring, New Delhi - 110 041
Tel. : 2557 5007 & 2568 448

Indian Cancer Society.
Q5A Jangpur Extension, New Delhi - 110 014
Tel. : 2431 9572, Fax : 2431 5785

Vimal Kamath
106, Dafodil, Palihill, Bandra, Mumbai - 400 050
Tel : 2605 6899

"HITAISHINI"
CD-54, Salt Lake, Sector-1, Kolkata - 700 064
Tel : 2337 5817

IRELAND :

The Irish Cancer Society.
URL: http://www.irishcancer.ie/

Women's Cancer Information Project.
URL: http://www.eurohealth.ie/cancom/index.htm

ITALY :

Lega Italiana per la Lotta contro Tumori - Italian League for fight against Cancer.
URL: http://www.legatumori.it/

UNITED KINGDOM :

Imperial Cancer Research Fund (ICRF)
URL: http://www.icnet.uk/research/index.html

Breast Cancer Care.
Central Office, Kiln House, 210 New Kings Road, London, SW6 4NZ.
Tel... 020 7384 2984.
Fax... 020 7384 3387
Email: bcc@breastcancercare.org.uk
Breast Cancer Care Help Line... 0808 800 6000

Cancer Link.
11 - 12 Northdown Street, London, N1 9BN.
Free Phone Cancer Link — 0808 808 0000
Self-help and support groups — 020 7520 2603
Email: cancerlink@cancerlink.org.uk

Cancer BACAP.
3 Bath Place, Rivington Street, London, EC2A 3JR.
Tel... 020 7696 9003 (Office)
Cancer Information Service — 020 7613 2121 (London) ;
Free phone 0808 800 1234 (out side London).
Web site: www.cancerbacup.org.uk

Break Through Breast Cancer.
Tel. 020 7405 5111.
Web site: www.breakthrough.org.uk

MacMillan Cancer Relief.
Tel. 0808 808 2020
Web site: www.macmillan.org.uk

Lymphoedema Support Network.
Tel. 020 7351 4480
Web site: www.lymphoedema.org/lsh

Cancer Research UK.
Tel. 0800 226 237
Web site: www.cancerresearchuk.org

INTERNATIONAL :

International Cancer Information Services.
URL:http://imsdd.meb.uni-bonn.de/cancernet/600299.html

GLOSSARY

103